TOPICS IN COMMUNITY HEALTH Series

BRITISH ASIANS – HEALTH IN THE COMMUNITY

PATIENCE KARSERAS SRN HV
Health Visitor, Cardiff
EIRWEN HOPKINS BA SRN RSCN SCM HV
Health Visitor, Cardiff

An H M + M Nursing Publication

JOHN WILEY & SONS
Chichester · New York · Brisbane · Toronto · Singapore

H M + M Publishers is an imprint of John Wiley & Sons Ltd,
Baffins Lane, Chichester, Sussex, England

British Library Cataloguing in Publication Data:
Karseras, Patience
British Asians: health in the community.
— (Topics in community health).
1. Asians — Medical care — Great Britain
I. Title II. Hopkins, Eirwen
III. Series
362.8′4 RA485

ISBN 0 471 91034 1

Library of Congress Cataloging-in-Publication Data:
Karseras, Patience,
British Asians
(Topics in community health) (An HM+M nursing publication)
Includes index.
1. Asians — Health and hygiene — Great Britain.
2. Community health services — Great Britain.
I. Hopkins Eirwen. II. Title. III. Series.
IV. Series: An HM+M nursing publication. [DNLM:
1. Community Health Services — Great Britain.
2. Ethnic Groups — Great Britain. WA 546 FA1 H7b]
RA485.H66 1987 362.1′089914041 87–8308

ISBN 0 471 91034 1

Typeset by Inforum Ltd, Portsmouth
Printed and bound in Great Britain by Biddles Ltd, Guildford.

BRITISH ASIANS – HEALTH IN THE COMMUNITY

To our British Asian families,
in gratitude for all that they have taught us.

CONTENTS

	Preface	ix
	Acknowledgements	xiii
1	Lifestyles	1
2	Communications	20
3	Childbirth	35
4	Infancy	62
5	Childhood	87
6	The Forgotten Years – From Youth to Old Age	109
	Appendix 1 Suggested Scripts for Weaning Advice	128
	Appendix 2 Phonetically translated Phrases for Child Development Assessment	132
	Appendix 3 A Concise Guide to the Cultures of British Asians Originating from the Indian Subcontinent	136
	Index	141

PREFACE

Readers who take the trouble to read prefaces before diving into the main texts, know that authors use them, firstly, as devices for declaring the purity of their intentions, thus pre-empting any philosophical ambiguities and, secondly, as a means of offering precautionary apologies for any offence they may unwittingly give in the selection of topics, handling of material or the terminology used. As newcomers to the world of writing we see no reason to deviate from tradition.

A book dealing with the contentious issues of culture, ethnicity and health certainly needs to state its aims and its authors' motivation if it is to escape accusations of 'racism' from woolly, radical thinkers and 'woolly, radical thinking' from racists. Writing a book of this nature is like walking a tightrope on which an incautious step in one direction leads to the danger of treating our subjects as specimens viewed through a microscope – interestingly different and worthy of observation but defined only in static, stereotypical terms – but if we do not describe, generalise and categorise, we fall into the trap of failing to provide readers with the knowledge they seek, and become guilty of obfuscation.

We start from the premise that the racism experienced by ethnic minorities in the delivery of health care stems more from the ignorance of practitioners than from prejudice. If only workers with a knowledge of minority cultures could disseminate their expertise among their colleagues, unintentional racism which can be as damaging to the recipient as deliberate discrimination, would gradually disappear from the health service. We believe this to be wholly desirable, – justifying means which, admittedly, are open to the criticism that as with any book delving into group needs, due prominence may not be given to the needs of the individual. Only the reader can redress the balance by ensuring that her priority remains the provision of health care based on the personal requirements of the client.

Our interest in minority health studies began when we were catapulted from the security of the health visitor course into practices for which we were ill prepared. We had been educated in the health visiting of the majority, white population and our knowledge of ethnic minorities was based on two lecture periods devoted to the topic. Given the already overcrowded syllabus, it would have been impossible to attempt more than a brief introduction. Real learning began after qualification but knowledge that is gained in the field must be at the expense of the client. There is no doubt that in the early years of practice, our inadequacies in discerning and meeting health needs caused offence, confusion and distress to those we were employed to help. We soon discovered that colleagues in other health-care disciplines were working in a similar state of limbo and that our problems were being experienced by health workers in all parts of Britain. The cri de coeur for theoretical knowledge has been partially answered by the increasing volume of literature being produced on the subject of ethnic minorities and health. Some describe cultures, religions and perceptions of health, others adopt an aetiological approach to the health 'problems' of minority groups while the most recent aim to raise the level of racism awareness among health workers. All very necessary, but there remains a gap – how to translate theory into services which accord with the client's expectations and lifestyle, and enables the worker to respond to health needs effectively and appropriately. With the utmost presumption, this book tries to provide workers with the missing links.

Our guiding principle in the choice of terminology has been the desire not to cause offence. Admissable nomenclature is ephemeral and writers run the risk of using words which are currently in vogue but may in later years provoke criticism. Take the example of 'black' versus 'coloured' – until recently 'black' was used derogatorily, 'coloured' being preferred by those anxious to display their lack of racial prejudice; now the position is reversed, thanks to a newly-awakened pride in the cultural heritage of black people which has encouraged non-whites to proclaim their blackness even though their skin may be only a shade darker than their white brethren who are not white anyway but, as E M Forster put it, 'pinko-grey'. As we are writing about only a few sections of the black population it would be too much of a generalisation to refer to our subjects as 'black', instead, we use the term 'Asian' although we realise that this too, is a misnomer because not all people from that vast continent are covered by the book. If we are strictly correct we should be referring to 'people living in Britain who have originated from the Indian subcontinent' which could lead readers to misinterpret a wish to be precise for pedantic longwindedness. When possible, we do try to be more specific by ascribing religious denomination or original geographical locality. To act as a balance in offsetting any unintentional offence we use the term 'native' with its connotations of unsophisticated peasantry to describe those whose forbears have lived in Britain for several generations and who identify solely as 'British'. The label 'immigrant' has implications of not yet belonging and has acquired a note of disparagement, therefore we use it only in connection with those who have just completed the act of migration. When quoting other writers we use their terminology although it may not accord with our own definitions.

If finding acceptable labels has been difficult in a racial context, it has been no easier for matters of sex. No doubt we shall incur the wrath of some of our readers by referring to babies as 'he' but to spread the anger more evenly, we call all health workers 'she'. Not everyone likes the expression 'health worker' but it does cover the range of professions and occupations which provide health care in the community. Our sincere hope is that the superficial irritant of questionable terminology does not detract from the contents of the book.

An explanation is also necessary on the decision to limit the subjects of the book to those from the Indian subcontinent, an approach which may appear to be unjustifiably narrow when taking into account the number of different ethnic groups for whom Britain is home. By restricting the area of study we are able to achieve greater depth and give a more detailed insight into culture patterns and health needs than would be possible had we attempted a blanket cover of all minority groups. As it is, the peoples of the Indian subcontinent, although once briefly united under the British Empire, comprise a number of distinguishable ethnic groups and those whom we have selected because they form sizeable communities in Britain, represent three major religions, three nation states and at least eight different languages; more than enough for one volume.

Having made our apologies and excuses, there only remains an invitation for the reader to read on.

PATIENCE KARSERAS
EIRWEN HOPKINS
1987

ACKNOWLEDGEMENTS

We have been touched by the tremendous amount of help and encouragement given by so many people that we hesitate to single out individuals but we are especially indebted to the following:

Ennid Edwards and Sidonia Innocent – Nursing Officers
Beti Miller – Health Education Officer
Jonathan Sibert – Consultant paediatrician, who acted as midwife for this venture
– all employed by South Glamorgan Health Authority
A Roma Choudhury – Ethnic Minorities' Librarian – South Glamorgan
Hettie C Hopkins – for ironing out the wrinkles in our grammar and spelling
Our families – for their tolerance of the highs and lows that have accompanied the writing of this book
Health Centre colleagues, past and present – for allowing us to share their expertise and experience
South Glamorgan Health Authority – for awarding us the 1984 Nursing scholarship which enabled us to widen our horizons

PK
EH

ACKNOWLEDGEMENTS

[illegible]

Chapter 1

LIFESTYLES

Any attempt to describe an Asian lifestyle is fraught with difficulty. Comparable in size with Europe, the Indian subcontinent has given rise to peoples as disparate in their ethnicity as the Europeans and for this reason we need to examine the major migrant groups as separate entities. There are, however, some characteristics common to all immigrants which have an impact on health and well-being and here we shall begin by venturing some generalisations.

While there may be remnants of the pioneering spirit that motivated the empire-builders of the last century, the modern migrant leaves his country because he is dissatisfied with his lot. If his home-circumstances were favourable he would have no need to seek improvement. The majority of immigrants come from neither the richest nor the poorest sections of Asian society: typically, they are small farmers working their own land but unable to provide a living for every member of the family. For some villagers migration is a way of life and an essential part of the economy, their remittances home often exceeding the income from the annual harvest.

The main centres of emigration are the states of Gujarat and Punjab in India, the Sylhet district of Bangladesh, Mirpur and the North West Frontier areas of Pakistan, together with that part of the Punjab falling within Pakistani jurisdiction. These are some of the wealthiest and most fertile regions of their respective countries but they are also border territories with a legacy of bloodshed and insecurity. It is not surprising that when asked what they consider to be the best aspect of life in Britain, immigrants frequently cite political stability.

There is a discernible pattern to the process of migration which began in earnest after the Second World War. An acute labour shortage in Britain coincided with the bloody aftermath of partition and attracted large numbers of male workers.

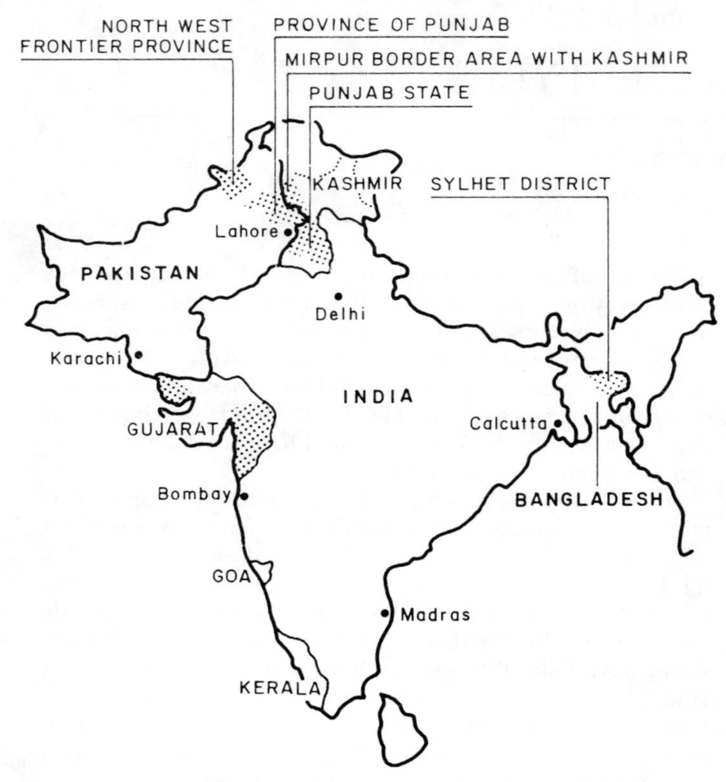

Fig. 1.1 Main emigration areas in the Indian subcontinent. (Reprinted from *Asian Patients in Hospital and at Home* by Alix Henley with the permission of King's Fund Publishing Office.)

Accommodation would be with fellow countrymen in all-male lodging houses. Work was uncongenial and usually on night shifts. Contact with native Britons was limited, with an unofficial but transparently obvious colour bar in operation. For their part, the immigrants viewed western society as decadent, irreligious and prejudiced, attitudes which are still held today. The only incentives to stay were high wages and loss of face had they returned prematurely. Most did intend returning when they could afford to retire and regarded themselves as sojourners rather than settlers (Ballard & Ballard 1877). The most pressing need was to amass sufficient funds in order that they could be reunited with wives and families.

Our concept of the western-style nuclear family, economically an independent unit, headed by parents who have selected each other as partners, and for whom religion is unlikely to be central to lifestyle, contrasts dramatically with Asian family life. Here, marriage unites families and not merely couples and, therefore, the choice of a suitable partner cannot be left to romantic whim but instead is entrusted to the wiser counsel of parents and elders. Children are the desired outcome of almost every marriage and failure to produce may result in divorce and subsequent disgrace for the woman. Families are usually joint (see Fig. 1.2), consisting of parents, sons, daughters-in-law, grandchildren and any unmarried daughters. When the father dies, the eldest son assumes the role of family leader. On marriage, a girl moves to her husband's home and only returns to her parental home for the birth of her first and, possibly, second child. The new wife looks to her mother-in-law and senior sisters-in-law for advice and instruction. In return, they share in the upbringing of her children who will relate equally to all the women of the house. Roles within the household are clearly defined; men and women work, eat and usually sleep separately, finding companionship with members of their own sex.

Maintaining such a lifestyle in Britain is almost impossible. Marriage partners have to make enormous adjustments both in their relationship with each other and in coming to terms with life in a cold, alien, urban society. Some of the older settlements are home to second and third generations but British housing rarely allows for the joint family to live under one roof. Many couples find themselves dependent upon each other for the first time in their lives.

The wife is probably the most disadvantaged, with little or no knowledge of English and even less of the complexities of an industrial society. Even if she does share a house with her compatriots there are still pressures. The average inner city house does not adapt well to the lifestyle of Asian families and, above all, the inhospitable climate precludes the outdoor life that could compensate for cramped quarters.

The husband, who may have lived in Britain for some years, could be presumed not to need any sympathy; after all, he

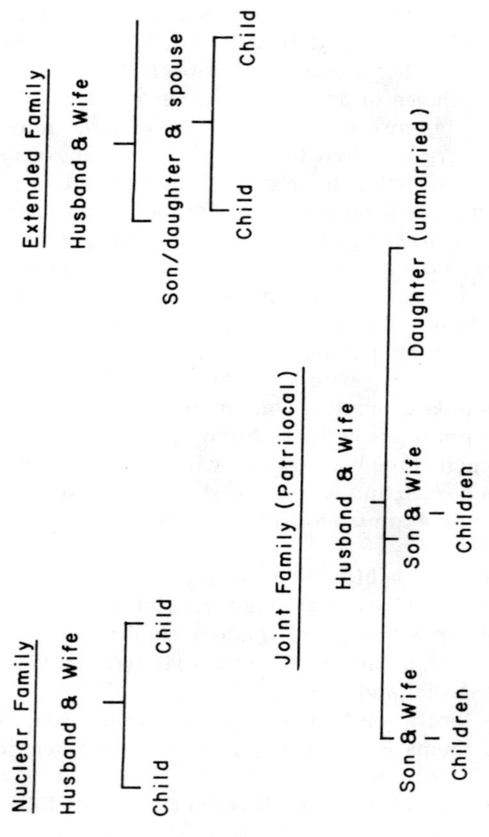

Fig. 1.2 Diagram to show different family structures.

speaks English, has his own friends and now that his wife is with him, he can expect more in the way of creature comforts. But he, too, has his problems. Financially, he has to set up a home and provide for his family because the chances are that unless he is newly-married, there will be children as well as a wife. He is expected to continue sending remittances home and at the same time, he is likely to be saving in order to start a business. His family will suffer from some degree of culture shock and he is the main source of emotional support. There is also the bureaucracy with which to contend: signing on with the doctor, applying for child benefit, enrolling the children at school and coping with bills for rates, heating, and so on, most of which will have been outside his experience when living as a single man in lodgings.

Almost all immigrants face insecurity, hardship and prejudice so it is not surprising that they seek out fellow countrymen and cling tenaciously to the 'old' life. The waves of people already absorbed into British society could all tell the same story. What has not been uniform is the level of integration, which has largely depended upon the actions of the immigrants and the reactions of the natives. The Jewish community who came as the result of religious persecution, have been assimilated into most areas of British life except those which clash with religious mores and here they have chosen to remain apart. Others, such as Polish refugees found it relatively easy to assume Britishness once the language barrier had been breached, unlike the Afro-Caribbeans who, despite similarities in religion and language, were, and still are, treated as outsiders because of their skin colour. If we assume that religion, language and skin pigmentation each play a part in shaping negative stereotypes and creating racial barriers, it is not hard to understand the difficulties confronting those newcomers who bring with them all three attributes and it goes some way to explain why Asians are now the prime targets for some of the ugliest manifestations of racism.

A common 'Asian' identity is formed by circumstances rather than any inherent similarities; it is now time to examine in more detail the different groups which comprise the Asian community in Britain.

Pakistanis

Those from the most northerly regions of the subcontinent are Pakistanis, peoples who in 1948 chose to form an Islamic state independent from the secular state of India. In appearance, they are tall and fair skinned, often lighter in colour than Europeans from Mediterranean countries. Dress for women is governed by a desire for modesty and consists of the shalwar and kameez, a pair of loose fitting trousers and knee length tunic. Also worn is the dupatta or chadar, a long scarf which is used to cover the face when the wearer is in the presence of men. The most orthodox Moslems, mainly those from the North-West Frontier, demand that, for their own protection, women are kept in Purdah and are secluded from all men other than close relatives. Women in Purdah never go out alone and even when accompanied by a husband, wear burqhahs, all enveloping garments with a small 'window' so that the wearer may see out but others are prevented from looking at her face. Daughters are expected to conform at puberty and from an early age have their legs covered with trousers or thick tights. Men usually wear western dress out of doors, sometimes with the addition of a brimless hat. At home, pajamas are worn.

Islam is central to lifestyle and governs every activity undertaken by its adherents. There are five specific duties: belief in Allah (God) and Mohammed, His Prophet; prayers must be said five times daily; fasting is to be carried out during the month of Ramzan (Ramadan); there are charitable obligations and, finally; once in a lifetime a pilgrimage must be made to the Holy City of Mecca. Islamic behaviour is learnt from the Holy Book, the Koran, which is taught to all children.

Often misunderstood is the status of women who, stereotypically, are seen as oppressed, with few rights and under the complete domination of husbands or fathers. In fact, Islamic women enjoyed a number of civil liberties including property rights and access to education, long before their western sisters. Within marriage, men are enjoined to be providers and protectors while women are responsible for the upbringing of children and household duties. Rahman (1980), quoting the Koran, describes the marital relationship thus:

> 'As human beings, women have equal rights with men: "Women have the same rights as husbands have over them in accordance with the generally known principles. Of course, men

(being active partners) are a degree above them (as seniors among equals)".'

For men, the focus of Islamic life is the Mosque. This may be anything from a room in a terraced house to a richly endowed, purpose built edifice straight out of *Sheherazade*. Women rarely go to the mosque but if they do attend, a separate room is used to keep the sexes segregated.

Diet is determined by religion. The pig is regarded as unclean and therefore not eaten. All other meat and poultry must be ritually slaughtered – Halal. (Several medium-sized towns in Britain have at least one Halal butcher). When circumstances force him to eat British food in, for example, school, hospital or works canteen, the orthodox Moslem will play safe and select a vegetarian menu. Some may find even this unacceptable because they cannot be certain that cooking utensils have not been contaminated with pork products.

Alcohol is forbidden but not tobacco. Women very rarely smoke but men are often heavy smokers.

The official language of Pakistan is Urdu which is spoken and read by educated people. The mother tongue is that of the locality and for those living in Britain, is likely to be one of the Punjabi dialects or Pushtu as spoken by those from the North West Frontier. Literacy rates are variable and it should not be taken for granted that adults are literate in their mother tongue, Urdu or English. The most commonly found combination is the ability to speak in mother tongue, to understand Urdu and for men, to read it as well.

Pakistani men prefer to be self-employed but initially take on any work in order to save for a business: the 'open all hours' corner shop, the 'chippie' and the one-man taxi service being typical examples. Women, unless they are among the educated minority, only go out to work if there are sufficient numbers to ensure all female Pakistani shifts. It is not the custom to work when children are young although many take in outwork for the garment trade and others help to run the family business.

Early marriage is favoured and girls are trained from a very young age in domestic skills and child care. Marriage is within a defined kinship group with first degree cousinship marriages not uncommon. The chosen partner may be British born, but many families like to strengthen the links with the subcontinent by selecting a spouse from 'home'.

Bangladeshis

Bangladeshis are also Moslems but they are distinguishable from Pakistanis by their shorter stature and darker skins. Women wear saris, using one end as a veil. Men wear western clothes when out of doors but prefer a 'lungi', a loose cotton skirt, for home use.

Edwin de H. Lobo (1978), describes Bangladeshi women as 'the sorriest, most downtrodden women in the world', basing this somewhat sweeping generalisation on a high suicide rate, short life expectancy, frequent pregnancies and the minimum of civil rights. These women do appear to be less assertive than their Pakistani sisters but whether this bears out de Lobo's assessment or is merely the result of culture shock, it is difficult to say. Bangladeshi families are the most recent settlers in Britain and are still in the early stages of adjustment. The men have been here for several years but for some reason have taken longer to bring over their dependents.

The first arrivals found work in Jewish clothing businesses in the East End of London and are today, the inheritors of the Brick Lane area, notorious for Fascist-inspired antisemitic riots during the thirties. Large numbers have moved out to the provinces where they are to be found in the restaurant trade. The Indian 'take-aways' are almost exclusively run by Bangladeshis although they would be the first to admit that the food produced is strictly for the western palate and bears little resemblance to any type of Asian domestic cuisine. The working hours of restaurant staff are barely compatible with family life so sensitivity is required from health workers when arranging home visits or clinic appointments.

It is not the custom for women to work and only well-educated, middle class women are to be found in employment. Parents are reluctant to allow their daughters to work on leaving school: they will probably assist their mothers until the inevitable early marriage.

Few of the women coming to Britain are able to speak English. The common language is Sylheti, a dialect of Bengali. Sylhet is the small area of North-east Bangladesh that is home for the majority of migrants. The official language is Bengali which is spoken and read by the educated minority and understood by most Sylhetis. Linguistically, geographically and politically, Bangladeshis are isolated from both native and Asian-born Britons. They do share a common religion with Pakistanis but memories of the bitter struggle for independence precludes amity between the two, erstwhile-united, peoples.

Dietary laws are similar to those observed by Pakistanis but because Bangladesh lies on the Ganges delta, fish is an important source of nutrients. In accordance with Islamic law, only fish with fins and scales may be eaten. Rice is also grown in the hot, wet climate whereas Pakistan is a wheat producer.

Gujaratis

The Gujarati community comes from two areas on the North-west coast of India. Approximately 10 per cent are Moslems but the majority are Hindus. Hinduism, as Bowker (1983) admits, is difficult to define: 'a coalition of many different teachings and practices'. The oldest of the Asian religions, Hinduism has no recorded founder and no set of doctrines. There are, however, priests, teachers and holy books to help the Hindu achieve his goal – unity with his Creator. Before he can hope for this, he must go through many cycles of birth, death and reincarnation, each life being determined by the deeds of the previous existence.

The concept of reincarnation helps us to understand the caste system which has dominated Indian life. A high-caste person has achieved his position because of his virtue in his most recent existence and is deemed worthy of higher regard than someone born into a lower caste whose former life was less perfect. The system is less rigid than in the past; the Indian government has outlawed the custom of untouchability which, for centuries had rendered the lowest caste, the Harijans, as outcastes. Increasing liberality in the subcontinent may have bypassed some of those who have lived in Britain for many years and can, in part, account for the wide social gulf between the high-caste doctor and his lowly-born patients.

The majority of Gujaratis come from one of the middle-ranking castes. There are further divisions into subcastes, based on locality and occupation. Marriages are always within the caste and usually between the members of the same sub-caste.

Prayer is an important part of Hinduism and it may be

conducted at home or at the Temple. Like Christianity, there are a number of sects, each with its own place of worship.

Dietary restrictions stem from a reverence for life. Many Hindus are vegetarian, relying on milk products, nuts and pulses to provide them with sufficient protein. Some do eat meat, but never beef because the cow is sacred and rarely pork because, like Moslems, they consider it to be unclean. Eggs are eaten by males but are considered unsuitable for women. Food is divided into two groups: 'hot' foods which include most of the protein-rich foods, thought to be stimulating and excitement-inducing, and 'cold' foods which have a calming effect and are, therefore, considered to be more suited to the passive ideal of womanhood. A careful balance is necessary to maintain an equilbrium and adjustments are made for pregnancy and illness.

Fasting is also included in religious observances: sometimes total abstinence is required but on other occasions, only certain foods are avoided.

The uninitiated may find it difficult to distinguish between the sari-clad women of Gujarat and their Bangladeshi sisters. The former are recognisable by their short blouses which leave the midrif bare. Another clue is the 'bindi', the coloured spot worn between the eyebrows of most married Hindu women. Some women colour the parting of their hair with a red paste. In appearance they are taller than Bangladeshis and, although valuing modesty, do not veil themselves. Many younger women, especially those born in Britain, adopt western trousers or long skirts. Most prefer clothes that cover the legs.

Hinduism places few constraints on integration, especially with regard to women who expect to work outside the home and will probably continue to do so after the arrival of children. Mothers-in-law, child minders and day nurseries are utilised to this end. Leaving aside racial disadvantage, employment aspirations for both men and women are similar to those of the natives, although owning a business is seen as highly desirable.

The spoken language is either Gujarati or Kutchi depending on the area of origin. Most understand Hindi which is the official language of India. Because there is a fair amount of contact with the natives most acquire sufficient English with which to cope, older women being the exception.

Indian Punjabis – Sikhs

Sikhism is an offshoot of the Hindu faith which developed in the sixteenth century when dissidents, led by the Guru Nanak, rebelled against the rigidity of Hinduism. Nevertheless, the two religions do have some beliefs in common, notably that of reincarnation.

The majority of Sikhs come from the Indian Punjab where demands for a separate Sikh state are being met with little success from the predominantly Hindu Government. Punjabi is the mother tongue but it differs slightly from that spoken by Pakistani Punjabis. The script is also different which has implications for health workers. Most Sikhs educated in India speak Hindi.

Traditionally, Sikh men have been adventurers. Many fought with the British during the Second World War and were respected for their bravery. Often at odds with the majority Hindu population, a number have emigrated and sought their fortunes elsewhere. Some have been extremely successful but for the average Sikh, life in Britain has been as much of a struggle as it is for all migrant groups.

Like their Pakistani neighbours, the women wear the shalwar and kameez but usually of a more ornate design. Make up and jewellery are commonly worn. The scarf, decorated with beads or gold and silver threads, is worn around the neck when indoors and covers the head when the wearer is in the presence of unrelated men. Men wear a turban over their long hair which must not be cut. Young boys have their hair pulled into a topknot which is covered by cotton material. Uncut hair is one of the five signs of Sikhism – the others are a comb worn under the turban, a sacred undergarment, a small dagger, and most importantly, a metal bangle which must always be worn. In order to reduce hostility from the natives, the first settlers abandoned the turban and cut their hair. Now, due to increased confidence, pressure from their womenfolk (always a force for religious conformity), and a worldwide rise in ethnic consciousness which has touched all migrant groups, Sikhism is displayed with pride.

Although Sikhs repudiate the caste system there are social divisions. Most British Sikhs come from the Jat caste, originally agrarian peoples who farmed smallholdings. Those coming via

East Africa are mainly Ramgarhias with a tradition of tie craftsmanship. The two groups do not intermarry. Employment patterns are similar to those of the Gujaratis, although it has been our experience that women are less likely to work when their children are small.

Sikhs observe fewer dietary prohibitions than Hindus although those who have made an extra commitment to their religion by participating in the ceremony of Amrit, promise to abstain from meat, fish, eggs, alcohol and tobacco. Lamb and poultry are acceptable to the majority but beef is not eaten, nor is the unfortunate, or perhaps fortunate, unclean pig! Fasting follows a similar pattern to Hindus but each religion has its own days set aside for this purpose.

Sunday is kept as a Holy day when Sikhs go to the temple (Gurdwara) which offers opportunities for corporate worship together with the facilities of a social centre. A meal prepared by the women is an integral part of Sunday at the Gurdwara.

East African Asians

Not all Asians have come to Britain direct from the subcontinent. Many migrated to the then British colonies in East Africa and became very successful in running the business life of their adopted countries.

Independence led to a policy of Africanisation with the forcible takeover of those businesses. Some decided to cut their losses and try their luck in Britain, others stayed on, only to be evicted wholesale from Uganda during the Amin regime. They fled to Britain as penniless refugees and suffered psychological and physical deprivation in addition to the usual traumas of migration. In their favour, they had had experience of living in an urban and cosmopolitan society including some knowledge of English and they were received with more sympathy and gestures of help than are accorded to those arriving through the normal channels.

The majority of East African Asians have their origins in Gujarat and the Punjab but because of caste and different backgrounds there is little contact with those coming direct from the subcontinent.

Naming Systems

We do not intend writing at length about naming systems which, unless learnt rather like multiplication tables, are guaranteed to throw officialdom into total confusion. We recommend the reader to the King's Fund booklet (Henley 1979) which sets out the different systems simply and clearly. Reducing the rules to basics, Moslem couples have different names as do their sons and daughters. Each person has a religious or titular name, a personal name and sometimes a family name. For example:

Husband	– Mohamed (religious) Azad (personal) Miah (family)
Wife	– Hamida (personal) Begum (titular)
Son	– Shafiq (personal) Ali (titular)
Daughter	– Salima (personal) Bibi (titular)

Gujarati Hindus have personal names, complementary names and subcaste names of which the most common is Patel. Some families are choosing to drop the subcaste name. Daughters use their father's complementary name until marriage when they adopt their husband's name. Sons may add their father's complementary name to their own when they reach adulthood.
For example:

Husband	– Vijay (personal) Das (complementary) Patel (subcaste)
Wife	– Indira (personal) Vijaydas (complementary) Patel
Son (14)	– Ravi (personal) Lal (complementary) Patel
Son (21)	– Anil Lal Vijaydas Patel
Daughter (7)	– Manjula Vijaydas Patel

All male Sikhs share a religious name – Singh – which means lion. Women take the name – Kaur or princess. To these are added a personal name and sometimes a subcaste name, both names being common to men and women.
For example:

Husband	– Amrit (personal) Singh (religious) Virdi (subcaste)
Wife	– Gurmeet (personal) Kaur (religious) Virdi (subcaste)

Son – Jaswant Singh Virdi
Daughter – Balvinder Kaur Virdi

A glance through any telephone directory will show that large numbers of Sikhs do not use their subcaste name, preferring to be known by their religious denominator, Singh.

We strongly advise readers to learn the naming systems and the commonly-used Asian names, as these will give immediate clues to a client's religion and country of origin and facilitate the planning of health care on reasonably accurate assumptions.

We must add a caveat born of our own experience. As the Asian communities become more familiar with western practices, learning the hard way just how hopeless we are at grasping the essentials, they adopt our system in which all members of one family share a common surname. Thus a Moslem wife will introduce herself as Mrs. Ali, the Sikh as Mrs. Singh. Alternatively, they may use the names which we have erroneously given them, such as Mr. Mohamed or Mrs. Begum. This is fine so long as everyone is happy and there is consistency when names are given for record keeping but what often happens is that clients name themselves according to their estimation of the official's level of knowledge. For example, to the Asian doctor, the patient will give the traditionally correct name which is also likely to be how he would choose to be called. To the health visitor, blessed with a little learning, the title could become a surname, while the uninitiated records clerk will have the entire family under one name. The best advice comes from Alix Henley (1979) whose suggestions are included in later chapters.

Leaders

When attempting to learn more about the ethnic minority groups in your area, you may follow the frequently proffered advice to 'seek out the leaders'. You may also find yourself getting nowhere, fast. The reasons for your difficulties are twofold. Firstly, the person who claims to represent a specific group and who sits on civic committees as their spokesman, may have a very different background from those he is deemed to lead. Typically, he is city bred and well-educated, perhaps with only a limited understanding of the problems facing 'his people'. Because of his social status he may be ambivalent about acknowledging that those problems exist. Secondly, just when you think you have identified the group and its leader, someone else appears also claiming to be the true leader. What you had assumed to be a single group actually consists of a number of sub-groups, each with its own spokesman – very confusing!

We suggest you look for the religious leaders, remembering that although they are not full-time professionals as in most Christian churches, they do know their 'flock' and are in a position of influence. Remember, too, that like Christianity, there are many branches of each faith and, hence, many leaders.

Areas of Britain with a well-established minority population are producing leaders from within the community. A few are women and they will prove invaluable to the health worker seeking to improve her services. In the main, women's interests come low down in the priorities of most leaders, and workers may find themselves lobbying for their female clients.

The head of the family should be identified. It is possible that he has stayed in the subcontinent. Nevertheless, he is consulted on a number of family matters including marriages and financial transactions. Those working with Bangladeshis should seek out the restaurant owners as they may be employing a number of compatriots and probably housing them as well. The owner's wife may take staff wives under her wing and because of her relative affluence and knowledge of the system she is an important source of advice and influence. One can find breast-fed babies attached to one restaurant and bottle feeders at another; it all depends on the preference of the boss's wife!

Housing

Asians tend to live in the older, more deprived areas of inner cities. Aspirations, like those of the natives, are for a nice house in a 'good' neighbourhood but with enough room for the extended family. For most immigrants the reality is less salubrious. Typically, there are several changes of address as families settle and become more prosperous. We have found that the newly-arrived family stays with an established person, often a relative, from their home village. Some addresses crop up time and time again and seem to be clearing houses with one permanent family plus a transient population of compatriots.

Length of stay varies but it is rarely longer than three months after which the family move on to the next address, usually, but not invariably, in the same district. Thereafter, much depends on the economic progress made by the immigrant and the type of housing available. The man who has been here for some years before sending for his wife and family may have amassed sufficient funds for house purchase in which case he can bypass the first two steps. It is more likely that a large proportion of his savings will have gone on travelling expenses. Some families apply for local authority housing and because they may be assessed as overcrowded in poor accommodation, should achieve priority status on the waiting list. Health workers should think twice before encouraging such a move. Most local authority housing is on large estates on the outskirts of conurbations. Rehoused families find themselves miles away from friends, specialist shops and religious centres. They may become the butt of local resentment and racial hostility. Others are offered a flat in a high rise block which, if accepted, would impose an even more drastic change of lifestyle for people who, before migration, invariably lived at ground floor level. At best, council accommodation offers a breathing space in tolerable surroundings at a reasonable rent: at worst, a nightmarish existence in which physical comforts can in no way compensate for isolation and constant fear of racist attacks.

When families are in a position to buy a house there is usually a pooling of resources with father, brothers or cousins buying a stake in the property. Not all the owners live in the house but they will take a share of any profits accruing from lettings. Workers should not assume that one family is the sole occupier and what we might judge to be overcrowding is as likely to occur in owner occupation as it is in rented housing. However, overcrowding is in the eye of the beholder and may actually improve the quality of life by providing extra cash and companionship for otherwise isolated families. Therefore, unless there are manifest health hazards or families themselves complain, the wisest course is to leave well alone.

Health workers frequently make assumptions of overcrowding on the basis of traditional Asian sleeping arrangements. A native family of parents and children sharing one bedroom would feel very hard done by but in the subcontinent it is considered unnatural and unkind to separate children into bedrooms of their own. Ideally, men and women sleep apart: the husband and older boys sharing one room while the wife, daughters and young children occupy another. Because most of the families visited by midwives and health visitors do have young children, they are likely to be together in one room with the youngest child sharing a bed with his mother. The husband may chose to forgo a room to himself in the interests of economy, joining the rest of the family in what appears to be a room in which every available inch of space is occupied by beds.

It is interesting to observe the change in native attitudes to taking babies into parental beds, a custom which, in the past was guaranteed to provoke critical comments from health workers. The late Hugh Jolly, renowned as a paediatrician, deserves credit for publicising the benefits for mother and baby but workers should also recognise that we have been influenced by cultures other than our own.

Home Visiting

Home visiting forms the bedrock of community nursing. Whether the worker visits to perform a specific task or, as in the case of the health visitor, to offer preventive health care based on assessment and health education, the relationship with clients is deeper and potentially more fragile than that arising from a clinic or hospital encounter. When visiting Asian families we have a role beyond that of health care provider. Although we are guests in our client's homes, we are also hosts with a duty to help newcomers to feel at ease and to acquire a sense of belonging. Health visitors may be the only regular visitors from the indigenous population and as such may be used as a yardstick by which western society is judged. Whatever the preconceived notions about native health workers may be, the Asian philosophy is that any visitor is to be honoured and treated with the utmost courtesy, no expense being spared to make her feel welcome. Previous unhappy encounters with officialdom may inject some apprehension as to the purpose of the visit, which should be explained as soon as possible.

This is jumping the gun because although the worker will indeed be treated as an honoured guest once the door has been opened, that same door may remain firmly closed despite the sounds of life emanating from the other side. The most likely reason is that the husband is out and the wife will not admit anyone unless she can be certain that the visitor is female. Having rung the bell it is advisable to stand back so that you may be scrutinised through a convenient window. Male doctors are regarded as a special case but any other category of male worker will only gain access if accompanied by a woman, preferably one known to the family. If referrals are made to other agencies it is worth making this point clear.

Workers should time their visits carefully. The three religions enjoy a number of festivals which combine religious observances with family reunions and celebrations. Needless to say, a visit from a health worker, unless medically essential, would be as welcome as one to a native on Christmas day.

Friday is not a good day to visit Moslems. It is equivalent to the Christian Sunday and although women do not go to the mosque, they do spend much of the day conducting their own private prayers. If you are visiting when prayers are due, you may be asked to wait until they have been said. Unlike those of the Christian faith, Moslems have no inhibitions about praying in front of others.

Ramzan, the Moslem month of fasting, also presents problems for the would be visitor. Adult members of the household fast during the daylight hours which, in the summer, entails considerable loss of sleep which is made up during the day (see Appendix 3). Prayers must also be said. Afternoon visits are usually safe but do avoid the morning.

Bangladeshis involved in the restaurant trade appreciate not being disturbed before late morning. When there are only pre-school children in the home it is customary for the whole family to adopt restaurant hours and to sleep between closing time in the early hours and lunch time opening. Again, afternoon visiting is best.

Asian hospitality will probably include the offer of a cup of tea. Opinions are divided as to the correct response. One school of thought believes that the offer should be accepted because a refusal causes deep offence. The holder of the opposing view who happens to have a weak bladder and has only recently acquired a liking for Indian-style tea, reckons that so long as gratitude is expressed, the health worker/client relationship will not be impaired if you say 'no'. For those unacquainted with Asian tea making, the leaves, water, milk, sugar and spices are brewed together to make a drink that is absolutely delicious but quite unlike the native 'cuppa' – definitely an acquired taste.

References

Ballard & Ballard R (1977) Between two cultures. In Watson J (ed) *The Sikhs*. Oxford: Blackwell

Bowker J (1983) *Worlds of Faith*. London: BBC/Ariel Books

Henley A (1979) *Asian Patients in Hospital and at Home*. London: King's Fund

Jolly H (1978) *Book of Child Care*. London: Allen & Unwin

Lobo E de H (1978) *Children of Immigrants to Britain*. London: Hodder & Stoughton

Rhaman A (1980) *Islam Ideology and the Way of Life*. Muslim Schools Trust

Recommended reading

Henley A (1983) *Asians in Britain Series*.
Caring for Moslems and their Families
Caring for Sikhs and their Families
Caring for Hindus and their Families
London: DHSS/King's Fund. Valuable background information with a health care perspective.

Chapter 2

COMMUNICATIONS

All health workers must be able to communicate with those they serve if they are to identify needs, agree on mutually acceptable means of action and achieve health enhancing goals. Although workers may experience frustration when the language barrier appears to be unbreachable, this is negligible when compared with the distress and anxiety suffered by the client. Unable to report a history or to describe symptoms, medical care for him must be a hit or miss affair, without benefit of explanation or reassurance. Compliance cannot be relied upon and therapy requiring patient participation will be useless and even dangerous because instructions are not understood.

At least clinical medicine offers tangible solutions to the relief of illness which are only partially dependant upon verbal interaction between client and therapist. In contrast, the health visiting service cannot be in the least bit effective in a non-verbal context. Its declared aims of promoting health and the prevention of ill health are achieved by education, suggestion and persuasion, all tailored to the client's perceptions, attitudes and goals. With health visiting, actions do not speak louder than words and communication skills which are essential to all health workers, must be honed to perfection if the health visitor is to make a positive contribution to the nation's health. This chapter examines ways by which all health workers can penetrate the language barrier.

Assessing the Client

Fluency levels are determined by a number of factors which include the age at migration; as a rule of thumb, the younger the immigrant, the easier it is to acquire a second language. Those who have experienced education, especially if the school taught in a medium other than their mother tongue, should manage a new language with less difficulty than their uneducated, monoglot peers. The best way to master a language is through regular contact with the natives, and here men and children have a clear advantage over their more isolated womenfolk. For women, opportunity and incentive often go hand in hand, as in the example of the wife who helps in the family shop, or the bride, recently arrived from the subcontinent, who joins a family in which the younger generation is bilingual, using English as often as their mother tongue.

How people learn and use a new language differs widely; workers should therefore avoid falling into the trap of making assumptions based on one or two encounters. Some Asians experience little difficulty in speaking English but become confused when they hear it spoken. Others, and our impression is that they are the majority, understand more than they are able to speak or are prepared to speak, given that confidence plays such a large part in the use of language. On a one-to-one basis, the client is likely to use her English to the limits of her ability but in the company of others more fluent than herself, she may fall back on her own language, preferring to use a companion as an interpreter.

Making Do

Very few people are totally non-English-speaking so it makes sense for workers to use what language there is in common. Words like 'doctor', 'hospital' and 'clinic' are invariably understood while 'nurse', 'baby' and 'husband' are known to most people. With these words it is possible to give a rough idea of identity and the reason for the contact. If this is at home the family may have contingency plans for dealing with officialdom such as a telephone number where the husband may be contacted or a friend living nearby who can be called upon to interpret. An evening visit is likely to be the most productive, but most health workers only undertake these as a last resort. If no headway is made, a note may be left, outlining the purpose of the visit, giving the time of the next one and requesting the presence of an English-speaker. Even if the husband is unable to read English himself, he will know someone who can act as a translator. Reading a second language that is handwritten can be difficult unless the writer omits personal idiosyncracies and reverts to the standard script beloved of primary school teachers.

Contact at this level is better than nothing but has little to recommend it. The use of a family member as an interpreter will inevitably inhibit the client from expressing her feelings. If her husband interprets, the woman will be conscious of his approval or lack of it, of what she is saying. He may not consider her anxieties worth passing on and, conversely, he may not consider it necessary for her to understand what is being said by the professional.

Children are often used as interpreters for non-English-speaking family members, a practice deplored by Rack (1982). The disadvantages include the reluctance of the mother to discuss intimate matters in front of her own child and if she does talk about her problems the woman places a heavy burden of knowledge upon the interpreting child who is likely to become insecure and over anxious. School attendance suffers if the child is kept at home to speak for the mother. The only benefits are that children are usually very honest, repeating word for word what has been said, and may also gain from any health education that takes place during the visit. On balance, we cannot endorse the use of child interpreters but, like all health visitors, have heaved sighs of relief when the household has included a chatty, English-educated youngster who can at least help to establish a working relationship with the family.

Professional Interpreters

Without skilled help, the health worker cannot expect even to be minimally effective: the most she can hope for is to become a friend of the family. If she is to carry out her professional role among non-English-speakers she needs tangible support from her employing authority.

The most obvious solution is to employ interpreters, and a health authority with a sizeable ethnic minority population who fails in this respect is simply ignoring needs. Some attempt to get by with volunteers mustered from the ranks of employees: this system rarely succeeds because it is dependent upon the client's needs coinciding with the working hours of the 'interpreter'. Mismatching of class and sex also reduce the effectiveness of such schemes, not uncommon examples being the male porter sent to interpret for the woman in labour and the junior hospital doctor who spends as much time interpreting as he does practising medicine. For the community health service with its relatively isolated workforce, paid interpreters are essential. Interpreting is a skill which requires complete mastery of at least two languages and a professional approach to what is an extremely sensitive role. As Shackman (1985) points out, there is no recognised training or career structure for interpreters, although there are a number of schemes where training programmes have been devised to meet local needs, some run by health authorities and others, in areas with a small population consisting of several language groups, have emanated from the community to serve clients using a variety of agencies.

Irrespective of the source of funding, health workers and interpreters also need to be trained in each other's roles if some of the commonly quoted problems are not to arise. One fear is that the interpreter will take over the health workers's role and stories abound of lengthy dialogues between client and interpreter with the worker reduced to third party status, unable to get a word in edgeways. This has not been our experience and should not occur if the interpreter has a clear idea of the worker's aims and objectives. A pre-session briefing is therefore essential. Sometimes the worker forgets that it is the client with whom she is communicating and directs her conversation to, instead of through, the interpreter.

The client may feel intimidated by the status of the interpreter if the latter comes from the educated, middle classes. Conversely, the interpreter may feel ashamed of what she considers to be the ignorance of her compatriot and will wish to demonstrate an understanding on the part of the client when perhaps it does not exist. The health worker with a knowledge of Asian cultures and social divisions should be able to pre-empt this. If, on the other hand, the interpreter has come from the same community as the client, there is the possibility that anxieties concerning intimate family matters may not be voiced in the presence of a peer: promises of confidentiality may not be believed. The client may also have ambivalent feelings about a woman of her own community taking on a role which could identify her with western culture. An unmarried interpreter could be perceived as unsuitable for the transmission of information on pregnancy, birth and anything remotely connected with sex.

Link Workers

A few health authorities have recognised the need for more than just an interpreting service and have taken on link workers in their maternity and paediatric units. As the name suggests, the aim is to bridge the gap between the impersonal and bureaucratic health services and the Asian communities and, ultimately, to improve the maternal and child health of groups who do not feature well, statistically. The role does include interpreting but there is also an element of outreach; explaining and encouraging the uptake of services, acting as escort to women who would not normally go out alone, and helping them to cope with the demands of being a patient. By unravelling the complexities of such disparate matters as claiming welfare rights, keeping an appointment for an ultrasound scan and turning a piece of paper decorated with hieroglyphics into a bottle of iron tablets, it is hoped to make the service more acceptable and consequently better used.

Although the first link workers were hospital-based, a number of schemes have developed in the community which offer the client a go-between service for coping with all the bureaucracies that inpinge on daily living. Community link workers operate through a combination of outreach and consumer demand: they are not employed to assist professionals, although those with whom they are in contact are enthusiastic supporters of their work.

Advocates

Health authority interpreting and link-worker schemes have been criticised for attempting to fit the client to a service which was designed to meet the needs of the articulate, white consumer and has failed to make the transition to todays' multicultural society in which all members are contributors via taxation, but only a privileged few actually have a say in how the service should be delivered. Advocacy schemes were devised in order that those who had not previously had a voice could be heard. The advocate, ideally coming from, and chosen by, the community she is to represent, like a lawyer, has only the interests of her client to consider. If health care practices threaten to violate cultural norms she will intercede on her client's behalf. For example, she could refuse an examination by a male doctor or exert pressure on hospital catering staff to provide meals that conform with religious dietary laws. Any racism, whether actual or implied, can be highlighted; an important part of advocacy being to raise the levels of racism awareness among those caring for her clients.

The first scheme of this kind was the Hackney Multi-ethnic Women's Health Project which focused much of its work on maternal and child health care in the Borough. Its success has encouraged other areas to produce their own schemes or to add an element of advocacy to existing link worker projects.

Not surprisingly, advocates have to cope with varying degrees of hostility from health care professionals who have been accustomed to almost total patient compliance. Those who ask questions, make demands or refuse treatment are labelled as 'difficult' and treated accordingly. There is also a sense of rejection in that what health workers have offered in good faith, has been refused by seemingly ungrateful patients and their advocates. Until health worker training courses become less colour-blind and monocultural in their appoach, advocates can expect a negative response.

Advocates must be absolutely certain that any requests made for culturally-acceptable health care are those of the client and do not stem from their own perceptions of what constitutes appropriate care. There is a danger that the advocate, linguistically more able and socially more aware than her client, may attempt to impose a set of values and expectations to which the client may not actually subscribe, with the result that the client becomes the vehicle for the advocate's demands and not the other way round, as originally intended.

Leaving aside the possible disadvantages, the response to advocacy should be positive; after all, if the NHS were to be a perfect institution there would be no need for advocates and their continued existence should encourage us to broaden our scope and eradicate those practices which, despite good intentions, have had such a deleterious effect on the well-being of minority groups. Health visitors, who have a large element of advocacy in their own roles, are well advised to seek out local advocates in order to plan realistic and acceptable health care for their clients.

Interpreters, link workers and advocates share the twin evils of chronic shortage of money and insecurity of job tenure. Most schemes are funded by 'soft' money; grants which run for a year or so, with no guarantee of renewal. This impermanence precludes forward planning and suggests a lack of commitment on the part of those holding the purse-strings. Health workers must be prepared to do battle to ensure the continuation of worthwhile schemes that are in danger of collapse because their grants have expired.

Joining The Ranks

A criticism frequently levelled at the NHS is its failure to employ staff from minority groups. Employers respond with a plea that if there were any applicants they would certainly be taken on. Why is it that the health care professions in general, and nursing in particular, appear to be so unattractive to potential Asian candidates?

Firstly, parents are reluctant to allow their daughters to enter a profession which requires its practitioners to have extremely close contact with members of the opposite sex. Nursing and modesty, as defined in Asian cultures, are almost incompatible. Secondly, nurses in the subcontinent are usually untrained women of low status and they form the role models for parents who, if their children are to have careers, will want 'something better'.

Thirdly, marriage is central to career planning. As we have seen, most girls marry young and are often mothers in their teens. The prospect of a training that continues into the early twenties is not acceptable to parents anxious to make a good match for their daughters.

Fourthly, prospective employees could be forgiven for assuming that career prospects are bleak for non-white workers. Mares (1985) describes the channelling of overseas, black nurses into low-status specialities, the likelihood of applicants being offered places on state enrolment courses instead of undertaking general nurse training, and the small number of black nurses occupying senior nurse posts. Lipsedge (1982) describes the typical hierarchy of white consultant, brown junior doctor and black nurse. Again, black doctors fill the otherwise unfillable posts in unglamorous specialties such as geriatrics.

Finally, there are fears that cultural beliefs will not be respected, particularly with regard to dress. Much publicity was given to the hospital which forbade the wearing of trousers by an Asian pupil nurse. Her prospective employers were found guilty of indirect discrimination and, as a result, the then General Nursing Council amended their regulations, allowing authorities to make their own rules. Most employers are now willing to concur with religious requirements on dress.

A public relations exercise is called for among Asian school-leavers to make the NHS an attractive proposition for employment. Attention should be drawn to those careers which do not offend against modesty norms such as pharmacy and occupational therapy. A few Asians are coming into health care and one hopes that their experience will encourage further recruitment. If this is to be achieved employers will need to demonstrate their commitment of equality of opportunity for all staff irrespective of ethnic origins.

Although communication difficulties would be eased considerably if more workers shared the same linguistic background as their clients, we should question the desirability of recruiting workers from minority groups in order that they may serve their own people. This smacks of ghettoism and is not conducive to a healthy, multiracial society. Nor is it good enough to employ a brown-skinned person and assume that she will be acceptable to all Asians. A comparison would be the appointment of a Swede living in Bombay to work solely with the resident white population.

Polyglot Health Workers

Should those who work with the minority communities learn some of the languages or, to be more realistic should they try? The authors admit to being failures in the second category. The British are notoriously poor linguists and health workers are no exception with, at best, 'O' level French and a smattering of restaurant Spanish. Those who are fluent in a second language have usually spent some time living abroad.

There is benefit to be gained from learning a few key phrases: these are very useful when seeking answers to the yes/no variety. Clients are always delighted that we have tried to master a few words: indeed, they are only too keen to teach us more. Workers in areas in which one language predominates should be offered lessons, although this may not be practical if the population includes all the Asian language groups. In this case, it makes sense to supply workers with phrase books so that they can at least communicate at a very basic level. We suggest Urdu and Hindi, which are almost the same when spoken, and Sylheti, as being the most useful languages to learn in a multilingual area.

Having accepted that the current batch of health workers are a lost cause as far as learning anything beyond the simplest of phrases goes, we could improve the standards of future employees by including Asian languages on the school curriculum. If schools teach German and Spanish, why not Urdu and Hindi, which, incidentally, are all part of the same Indo-European language group with more similarities than one might expect. Some GCE examination boards do offer Asian languages as subject choices but candidates are mainly from the groups for whom they are mother tongues.

Learning English as a Second Language

The most obvious solution to the communications barrier is for everyone to share a common language but this is an aim that has not received universal support. As we have seen, men and children learn of necessity but with relative ease and it is the inability of women to acquire even basic English that has occasioned hot debate in the forum of race relations. From the women's point of view there may be little incentive to learn. Her friends are fellow countrywomen, the language of the home will remain in the mother tongue while the children are young, and entertainment comes from own-language video films. Husbands may actively discourage the acquisition of English, fearing that if women master the language they may be tempted to emulate some of the presumed decadence of the natives. There is also concern that if English creeps into the home, their own culture will be diminished and eventually lost. The assumption is that encouragement to learn English is disguised pressure to become anglicised, a view shared by Anil Bajpai (1985), writing as vice-chairman of the National Association for Teaching English as a Second Language to Adults (NATESLA), who suggests that an expectation to learn English is the last straw for women already under immense pressure adapting to life in Britain. He also criticises the failure of ESL teachers to allow their pupils to decide their linguistic goals and suggests that the lack of interaction between teachers and the taught has led to a black/white power imbalance.

Although few would disagree with the need for sensitivity in approach on the part of teachers, and a breathing space before ESL tuition is offered to the immigrant, we should not deny the value of learning English, especially with regard to family health. The following examples illustrate the dangers that may arise when English is not understood: infant milk feeds may be made up incorrectly because instructions, written or verbal, are incomprehensible; diagnosis is almost impossible without a history or description of symptoms; hospital and clinic appointments may be missed because times and dates are confused; accidental poisoning is a distinct possibility if medicines are not taken in the correct dosages. Add to these the extra burden placed upon the husband who has to act as interpreter, escort and shopper in addition to his breadwinning role, the disadvantages to the school child in having a mother who cannot help with homework, the increasing isolation of the woman who remains in a time warp while her husband and children adopt more and more British customs, and the sum total is a family under stress. If consumer satisfaction is used as a yardstick to measure the desirability of teaching English, our experience should encourage those promoting ESL as we have yet to meet the Asian woman who regrets having learnt English.

The practical obstacles to learning English should not be overlooked. Most local education authorities run ESL classes but these are patronised by male immigrants, au pairs and foreign students. Few Asian women would feel comfortable in a mixed group such as this even if they could manage the journey and find someone to mind the children. Ladies only classes are sometimes held but numbers attending are low, especially in Moslem areas where purdah restrictions make it difficult for women to leave their homes. The alternative is home tuition, which is very expensive if paid tutors are used and difficult to organise on a voluntary basis. Despite this, many excellent schemes do exist, usually under the aegis of NATESLA. Good liaison between health workers and ESL tutors can result in joint projects such as English for Pregnancy classes which are held in several parts of the country. The common experience is that tuition has to start in the home; later, when the confidence of the women and their families has been gained, small community-based classes do succeed.

ESL for Health Workers

ESL tutors rarely speak the language of their pupils and have to develop communication skills in order to make themselves understood, skills which would also be of benefit to health workers. One has only to listen to the euphemisms, jargon and idiomatic phrases that are the stock in trade of so many professionals to realise that we need educating in ESL techniques as much as our clients. If it is impossible for workers to attend classes they would do well to fall back on the invaluable advice offered by Alix Henley (1979). She decries the use of pidgin English but does advocate language devoid of frills when communicating with clients with a limited knowledge of English. Ensuring that you have been understood is essential; reliance on 'yes' or 'no' is too uncertain. If in doubt, the client should be asked to repeat the instructions/advice.

Body language is an essential adjunct to verbal communication. A spoken greeting without a handshake, salute or smile signifies very little. Facial expression, use of hands and tone of voice say as much about ourselves as our actual speech content. We tend to use body language unconsciously, more as a means of self-expression than a deliberate attempt to make ourselves better understood, but if it is to be used as a substitute for the spoken word it must be used explicitly. The comic example of the Englishman trying to direct the foreign visitor by raising his voice and waving his arms about is funny because it is so true to life.

At a clinic the client's co-operation can be gained by non-verbal means for a number of simple procedures such as weighing, removing clothes and estimating blood pressure. Approval should be indicated when the desired action has been accomplished and when appropriate, reassurance given that the result is satisfactory. The addition of simple words such as 'come', 'thank you', 'good' and 'okay' will add emphasis. If the words are not understood, voice tone will be, and there is something rather eerie about dealing with a client in total silence.

Culture and Language

The way in which we use a second language depends to a certain extent on how we use the mother tongue, and the hybrid resulting from this match has provided comedians with material for centuries. Sadly, in 'real' life, an imperfectly-used language is as likely to cause offence as it is to provoke laughter. Health workers with a knowledge of their clients' linguistic background may have to defuse confrontations between client and other health workers who have been offended by what they deem to be rudeness. The classic example is the patient who demands to see the doctor: the worker reacts to an abruptness of speech style and the absence of a 'please' by giving an equally curt retort, the patient becomes confused and angry and racial harmony bites the dust. If the worker had previously heard the person speaking in his own language she might have recognised a similarity and realised that the natural pattern of speech has carried over to his use of English. 'Please' and 'thank you' are not used in Asian languages; courtesy is implied in the words used and in the sentence construction. Unless the speaker has been taught that these words are a necessary part of English, it is unlikely that he will use them.

Body language is also culture-dependent and workers are often disconcerted by the lack of eye contact with their Asian clients. To the westerner, the steady gaze denotes a frank and honest person but to the Asian it indicates boldness and presumptuousness and is quite alien to their cherished values of modesty and humility.

The Written Word

Illiteracy is a serious handicap in a world which places great value on the ability to read. Those who emigrated to Britain in adulthood vary considerably in their literacy skills, with a sizeable minority being unable to read either their own language or English. As a generalisation, men, having received more education than women, are more likely to be literate but not necessarily in their mother tongue; for example, Bangladeshis speak Sylheti but are educated in Bengali while Punjabi-speaking Pakistanis are taught in Urdu. Those who have had the advantage of higher education can also read and write in English.

Given that the majority of men and women do read their own language, there are opportunities for the use of health education literature, and much painstaking work has gone into devising appropriate material. Sadly, most of it has not been worth the effort: the standard of translation is often poor and the advice given at odds with cultural practices. Some, in particular the Health Education Council's publications, are excellent, with clear, accurate scripts backed up by pictures which offer some guidance to non-readers. Before issuing leaflets, workers should check their contents with a translator and any deficiencies can then be passed on to the producers for rectification.

Teaching Aids

Increasingly sophisticated material is available to the health worker wishing to maximise her potential as an educator. A number of clinics and health centres have video recorders with a bewilderingly large choice of films all offering enlightenment to the viewer. The Asian population has not been neglected and Asian-language films may be had from a variety of sources. Some are produced by manufacturers, notably those making baby foods and equipment and their use does pose an ethical dilemma for the health worker, irrespective of the cultural origins of the audience because, no matter how valid the message, there is, even if only contained in the credits, an element of product promotion which the worker showing the film could appear to be endorsing. An English-speaking audience can be reassured of the worker's objectivity if she gives additional information on other available products but this is impossible if the audience does not speak English. Unless an interpreter can be present, such films are best avoided.

Locally-made videotapes are ideal but only for those in the locality in which they were made. Producing a videotape is expensive and in a rapidly changing climate of health care provision it should be borne in mind that such tapes could become out of date within a few years.

As with literature, the best videotapes are those made by agencies concerned wholly with the promotion of health. The advantage of videotapes over ciné-films is that they can be shown in the client's home provided there is a video recorder and these are to be found in the homes of most Asian families.

A cheaper alternative to the videotape is an audiotape recorded in the appropriate language, with relevant visual aids such as leaflets or flannelgraphs. Unlike videotapes, only the minimum of technical knowledge is necessary for recording on audiotapes so these can be produced by health workers to suit the linguistic needs of their local population.

The Mass Media

Health educationists recognise the powerful influence of the media in communicating messages about health to the widest possible audience, and use advertising space, publish articles and contribute to programmes devoted to health topics. Non-English speakers are unable to benefit from this type of education which is targeted at the mainstream, white audience, but they are compensated by the existence of own-language newspapers, television and radio programmes which all have potential for promoting health. The BBC Asian magazine programmes are popular with families and items on health appear to be well received. For obvious reasons, listening to the radio other than for its musical output is uncommon but community-based local radio has been used to good effect especially when publicising local initiatives or offering a 'phone-in' service.

Finally, we should not ignore the contribution of public libraries which are opening sections of literature written in the Asian languages. Although intended principally for recreation, libraries do have reference sections and are a focal point for advertising local facilities including those connected with health.

References

Bajpai A (1985) A new face. *NATESLA News*, No 21, 1

Henley A (1979) *Asian Patients in Hospital and at Home*. London: King's Fund.

Lipsedge M & Littlewood R (1981) *Aliens and Alienists*. Harmondsworth: Pelican Books

Rack P (1982) *Race, Culture and Mental Disorder*. London: Tavistock Publications

Shackman J (1984) *The Right to be Understood*. National Extension College.

Recommended Reading

Henley A (1979) *Asian Patients in Hospital and at Home.* London: King's Fund. Valuable advice contained in chapters on language and communication.

Mares P, Henley A & Baxter C (1985) *Health Care in Multiracial Britain.* Cambridge: National Extension College/Health Education Council. Chapter on communication

Shackman J (1984) *The Right to be Understood.* National Extension College. Essential reading for anyone working with interpreters.

Chapter 3

CHILDBIRTH

Perinatal mortality statistics are second only to death rates in demonstrating the health status of a specific population group. British Asians have yet to reach old age in sufficient numbers to make death rates statistically meaningful and, thus, all data on childbirth are studied with keen interest by those concerned with the health of this most recently arrived section of society.

Country of birth of mother	*1978*	*1982*
Bangladesh/India	21.3	13.85
Pakistan	24.9	20.1
All U.K. Births	15.1	10.9

Table 3.1 Perinatal mortality rates per thousand live and still births

Source: O P C S (Crown copyright. Reproduced with the permission of the Controller of Her Majesty's Stationery Office).

Although the decline in perinatal mortality rates have benefitted Asians and natives in roughly the same proportion, the disparity between the groups remains as wide as ever and this must provoke grave concern among professionals responsible for providing maternity services. The reasons postulated for this disparity include poor uptake of services, short intervals between pregnancies, grand multiparity, very old mothers, very young mothers, poor maternal health, low income, poor housing, intermarriage and failure to cope with contraception, with the implication that ethnic minorities must change their way of life in order to benefit from the bounty of our health care system: put simply, it is their fault. Only recently have workers begun to question the appropriateness of available services and to ask whether it is we, the health professionals, who need to adapt. This chapter examines how East and West can achieve compatibility in the sphere of pregnancy and childbirth.

Birth in the Subcontinent

The contrast between birth in Britain and in the subcontinent could not be more marked; only the common aim of a healthy, normal baby unites two very different means to the same end.

Pregnancy is the desired outcome of almost every Asian marriage. The inability to have children is not only a personal sadness for the couple concerned but also a tragedy for the entire family: thus, the newly-pregnant wife finds that her status is instantly enhanced. Antenatally, she is looked after by the women of the joint family who cosset her and prepare special food. She is primed for a life-threatening ordeal in which the only skilled help is likely to come from the village midwife who may be experienced but has had no formal training. Many women return to their own families for the birth, rejoining the marital home after the puerperium.

During her lying-in the new mother is expected to rest, keeping her energies for breast feeding which also demands the provision of a special diet. For some women it is customary to wait until the milk 'comes in' before putting the baby to the breast. Colostrum is considered too 'strong' and could cause the baby to choke. Sugar water is given instead for the first two or three days.

The recovery period lasts for about six weeks, after which a ritual cleansing bath is taken by the mother before she returns to normal household duties. The support and expertise of her female in-laws enables the transition from wife to mother to be made with relative ease.

Husbands are not involved in any aspect of care but they are expected to carry out the customary rituals of their religion. A Hindu baby is bathed according to ritual and then shown to the father who places honey and ghee on the tongue. The Moslem baby must have a call to prayer whispered into his ear as soon as possible after the birth. If the father cannot be present a male relative may perform this task. Sikh babies also receive special prayers. Couples avoid sexual intercourse during the lying-in period.

The British Experience

In Britain, the typical pregnant Asian woman looks to her

husband for support, knowing that her female relatives are struggling to manage their own immediate family commitments. Considerable adjustments have to be made in the marital relationship, which is already stressed with the complexities of life in western society. Pregnancy introduces the couple to unfamiliar areas of bureaucracy: filling in forms becomes a way of life. There are, seemingly, interminable visits to antenatal clinics where efficiency and effective medical care may be at the expense of cherished cultural values. Intimate personal details are elicited, often with the husband acting as interpreter. Women may be subjected to the indignity of a vaginal examination carried out by a male doctor accompanied, perhaps, by a number of male medical students.

The birth will almost certainly take place in the unfamiliar surroundings of a hospital labour ward where mothers are taken over by a system which monitors, mechanises and medicalises what had previously been looked upon as a natural event. Breast-feeding mothers are encouraged to suckle their babies immediately after delivery to stimulate lactation. Colostrum is valued for conferring immunity to the baby and a refusal to breast feed at this stage may be misunderstood as a wish to bottle feed with formula milks being given at feed times.

Hospital stays are brief. An average of five days for an uncomplicated first delivery and 48 hours for multiparous women are ordeals long enough for women unfamiliar with the routine orientation and lack of personal privacy that typifies most postnatal wards. Food is unpalatable and probably contravenes religious mores. A few hospitals have introduced menus which accord with the requirements, both in content and preparation, of the major Asian religions. A few more combine facilities for Jewish and Asian patients which meets some but not all needs. The remainder fall back on western-style vegetarian food which has not proved popular with Asian patients. The alternative is food prepared at home and brought in, a practice which is the norm for hospital patients in the subcontinent but which is viewed with mixed feelings by staff and other patients in British hospitals and may add to the burden of discomfort already suffered by the recipient.

Hospital hygiene arrangements may be bewildering to women for whom personal cleanliness is part of religious observance. The native custom of almost total immersion in a bath of water which is also used to wash all parts of the body, is regarded as being rather revolting. Showers and bidets are preferred.

Early discharge leads to the immediate resumption of household duties, including cooking, a task not normally undertaken at a time when women are considered to be unclean. Family circumstances vary considerably but very few women are able to enjoy a lying-in as described in the previous section; even if they could, health workers would impose expectations of early ambulation, exercise and clinic attendance.

Consumer Variations

Not all Asian women find British health care alien. The daughters of those who immigrated in the fifties and sixties are now of childbearing age and they share broadly similar expectations of maternity services as their native neighbours. Adjustments have to be made with regard to diet and other religious norms but meeting needs which can be articulated is relatively easy, provided that mothers are given the opportunity to express those needs. Too often, treatment is based on the false assumptions of the care givers who have not taken the trouble to assess the individual needs of their patients. Women are reluctant to make demands and are aware that a request for something which is not part of the standard provision is often perceived as an implied criticism. Thus, only the most assertive women are prepared to speak out. This was well illustrated by an obstetrician who stated that only middle-class Asian women objected to being examined by a male doctor, the rest seeming happy with either sex.

There is one group of Asian women who seem only too anxious to conform to all the norms of western patient behaviour: these are the ladies who have experienced traumatic deliveries, perhaps resulting in perinatal death, whilst living in the subcontinent. For them, the health service offers hope and they are prepared to tolerate any indignity in order to achieve their longed-for babies.

Most primigravidae are regular clinic attenders. Their husbands, not under pressure from other children, are usually in attendance and appear anxious that their wives should benefit from all aspects of care. When this group have had safe deliveries, the pattern for further pregnancies may differ, with couples seemingly less motivated: he, because he is now financially stretched with children to provide for, cannot take time off from work; she, having found her first delivery to have been a harrowing experience, will be only too happy to limit her contacts with the health service to what she defines as the absolute minimum for safety.

Also likely to view British maternity services with scepticism are those multiparous women who have recently been reunited with their husbands after years of living in the subcontinent. Having had successful outcomes to their previous pregnancies, they cannot understand why we make such a fuss and, finding that the system conflicts with all their values, decide to let nature take its course, unaided by modern medicine, until labour commences or things start to go wrong.

Current Antenatal Provision

Antenatal care starts with a visit to the general practitioner who will confirm the pregnancy. Thereafter, care is given in a bewildering variety of ways. Almost every confinement takes place in a consultant-based obstetric unit, with a small minority using a GP-run delivery unit and an even smaller number of low-risk women being 'allowed' a home confinement. Asian women, usually categorised as high risk, as demonstrated in Table 3.1 are generally booked for a hospital delivery. Antenatal care can be given wholly by the hospital or on a shared basis between hospital and GP. The attractions of the latter are familiarity, less travelling and shorter waiting times, but a study in Tower Hamlets showed that Bangladeshi women were more likely to attend hospital-only clinics than native and English-speaking immigrants (Watson 1984).

Variations are to be found in services offered by GPs. Some see antenatal patients during routine surgery hours, others hold separate clinics with midwives, health visitors and interpreters in attendance. The benefits of a specific antenatal clinic are continuity of staff and provision of services tailored to meet the needs of a small, local group of patients.

The converse of constantly changing staff and general inflexibility need not characterise the hospital antenatal clinic, although it often does. The presence of link workers can be very reassuring, especially if they are already known to the mothers. The Save The Children Fund's Asian Mother And Baby Campaign has sponsored a number of link worker schemes and although these have been criticised, for reasons explained in Chapter 2, experience suggests that mothers are very appreciative of the services.

Clinic visits entail a certain amount of form-filling which, without the aid of an interpreter, can be frustrating for worker and mother alike. The first stumbling block is how to record the mothers' name correctly. As we have seen, naming systems can confound the uninitiated. If possible, the name given should be cross checked with the name on the woman's medical record, which should also carry the name of her husband. Then the worker can ask the woman how she would like to be addressed: for example, would she prefer Nassia Khatoon, Mrs. Khatoon, Mrs. Meah or Nassia Meah? Most will opt for the style of Nassia Khatoon, which is the accepted form of address in the subcontinent and the preference should be recorded.

It is not always possible to ascertain the exact date of the mother's birth because that recorded on passports and official documents could have been devised to satisfy the authorities and in some instances, can be wrong by as much as a decade. It is better to specify that the exact date is not known than to copy a spurious one – at least the obstetric team will not be lulled into thinking they are caring for a woman younger or older than she really is. On the other hand, because of their religious significance, menstruation dates are usually remembered and can be relied upon for accuracy.

Women unable to write in English are often uncomfortable when asked to sign their name. Reassurance that signatures in their own script, or marked with a cross, are legally valid always brings relief.

Home Visiting

Health visitors need to establish contact with the expectant family as soon as possible. Taking services to the client is part of the concept of 'outreach' and is a departure from the 'take it or leave it – at your peril' philosophy which typifies so much clinical health care. Health visitors have always pursued their own brand of outreach, enshrined in *An Investigation into the*

Principles of Health Visiting (CETHV 1977) as the search for health needs. Home visiting during the antenatal period is where the search begins.

Privacy enables fears to be expressed and questions to be asked which might remain unvoiced in a clinic setting where the lack of time and space imposes inhibitions. In her own environment the mother can be herself and can enjoy an equal relationship with the worker which is impossible in a clinic where she has neither the professional skills needed for her own welfare nor the territorial advantage of being on home ground.

Although health visitors resent the accusation that they are 'nosy', it would be hypocritical not to admit that the mother's lifestyle as seen in her material surroundings, does form part of the assessment made on the likely health visiting needs after the baby is born. Of far greater importance are the mother's attitudes, values and perceived needs, and the relationship she has with those who share her life. Indeed, one cannot fully know the Asian woman without meeting her family. While the mother is certainly an individual in her own right, she is also an integral part of a family group with its own identity, even though all its members may not live under her roof.

As in all families, conflict may arise and not all members are in complete harmony with each other. Often it is the daughter-in-law who feels set apart from the others. Marriages are arranged with the compatibility of the uniting families as one of their criteria but dissimilar backgrounds can give rise to differing expectations, a typical example being a match between a girl who has been brought up in the subcontinent and a boy with a British education whose family have acquired a western outlook on life. Here, the new wife may be scorned for her lack of sophistication while she is perhaps shocked at some of the family's western habits. Conversely, the British-educated Asian girl who marries into a family only recently arrived from the subcontinent, may find that her western ways incur disapproval and that freedoms, hitherto taken for granted, may be curtailed. Pregnancy, while being welcomed by all the family, can accentuate differences and increase tensions. Fortunately, these examples form only a small minority but when they do occur, a health worker willing to lend a listening ear can be a source of valuable support.

The antenatal visit is likely to be the first home visit from a health worker other than the GP and unless the purpose of the visit is immediately made known, there may be fears that the worker is 'checking up' on the family. For this reason it is best not to take down any written information about the family and questions should not be too specific. A polite interest in the family's length of stay in Britain could be misinterpreted as querying the legality of their citizenship and questions about the country of origin may be perceived as racially motivated. Anyway, the well-educated health worker has no need to ask such questions. She will recognise the religious background from the style of dress and can discern from the accent whether the speaker was brought up locally, in another part of Britain or in the subcontinent.

The woman who is part of an extended or joint family does not remove herself from the company of her female relatives for the visit, so there may be no opportunity to speak to her alone. However, subjects such as breast feeding, which native women might prefer not to discuss in front of others, are acceptable and, remembering the degree of influence exerted by the family, more suited to a wider audience. Couples are not easily seen apart from the family other than in their bedroom. Space permitting, the women occupy one living room, their menfolk another. Ironically, for a number of prospective parents the only opportunity for a private chat with the health workers is at the clinic.

Closing The Gap

By becoming more approachable, adapting the services to conform with differing cultural values and by pursuing a policy of outreach, health workers may help to build a span or two for the bridge that could close the gap between native and Asian perinatal mortality rates. Other statistical determinants are harder to change.

Racial disadvantage places most black immigrants near the lower end of the social scale. Black (1982) has described how those in Social classes IV and V (Registrar General) suffer inequalities in health care, and that poor social conditions contribute to ill health, lower life expectency and more lost babies. The Inverse Care Law states that those with the greatest health needs obtain the least in the way of health services (Hart 1971).

The adverse effects of social inequality on the health of Asians in Britain are born out by a study in Peterborough which showed that perinatal mortality rates were the same for native and Asian populations (Dryburgh 1985). Peterborough cannot have been uppermost in the minds of Black and Hart as they pondered the results of deprivation. As a city, it is not noted for poverty or urban decay and their concomitant social problems, as are London, Liverpool and Birmingham. The quality of life for its citizens must be as good as that offered by any other medium-sized conurbation in Britain.

The purpose of the study was to find out why Asian babies were lost at birth and the results show that Asian and native babies die for different reasons. Native babies die mainly from the effects of prematurity whereas lost Asian babies were carried to term but were light for dates with evidence of intra-uterine growth retardation. Death from malformation was also significantly higher than for native babies.

Poor nutrition is believed to be a major cause of intra-uterine growth retardation (IUGR) and claims that women in Birmingham eat less well than those in Islamabad are disquieting (Wharton 1982). Asian diets, if correctly balanced, can provide all the nutrients for health, and in many respects, are superior to the high-fat, low-fibre, additive-ridden food consumed in the west. Availability of Asian foods is not usually a problem but prices may be high, reflecting the cost of importation (see page 47 for dietary advice).

Consanguineous marriages have also been implicated in the high incidence of IUGR (Sibert 1979). Intermarriage within the kinship group is common in several areas of the subcontinent and history-taking should always include an enquiry about whether there is a blood relationship between husband and wife. The risk of congenital abnormalities is also increased and there is a greater chance of offspring being affected by inherited disorders such as thalassaemia, in which the condition occurs only when both parents are carriers with a one-in-four chance of an affected offspring. Ideally, the woman should be screened preconceptually and if the result is positive, screening should then be offered to her husband. If both parents are known to carry the trait, fetal screening at nine weeks' gestation can predict whether the disease is present with reasonable accuracy and parents then have the option of an early termination of pregnancy. Parents tested during the mother's pregnancy can still be offered prenatal screening at 18 weeks' gestation, the disadvantage being the trauma associated with a late abortion. All medical intervention needs to be accompanied by sympathetic and informed counselling. Drop-in centres exist in a few major cities and offer screening, information and counselling on thalassaemia, sickle cell disease and other less severe haemoglobinopathies which have been a major cause of early death and ill health in those originating from the warmest regions of the world.

Genetic counselling on the risks of inherited diseases in consanguinous marriages may be perceived as an attack on a custom that has been an integral part of Asian cultures for centuries and, indirectly, as an attempt to destroy the culture, but if they are to make an informed decision couples cannot have information withheld because the worker is afraid of causing offence.

Intestinal Parasites

The woman who has recently been in the subcontinent may present with a low haemoglobin level and abdominal discomfort. A stool specimen should confirm a diagnosis of roundworm or hookworm infestation. This is a common condition in hot countries and although the effects are relatively minor in most instances, parasites do reduce feelings of well-being and can exacerbate any existing problems associated with nutrition. Treatment is simple and effective and should be given to all members of the family. Although infestation can occur at any time, it is only during pregnancy that haemoglobin is routinely checked and general health so carefully monitored.

Preparation for Parenthood

The British approach to childbirth can be summarised thus: a woman who has prepared herself physically and mentally for the birth of her child, and who knows and understands how her body functions during pregnancy and labour, is more likely to produce a healthy infant in atraumatic circumstances than the woman who adopts an ostrich-like posture and 'does not want to know'. Because communication barriers appear unbreachable, health workers erroneously assume that Asian women fall into the 'ostrich' category. On the contrary, they are as avid for knowledge as any other group of pregnant women but do not consider that the standard parentcraft training as taught to native mothers is culturally acceptable. Some girls, sent to classes at the behest of their westernised husbands or over-zealous health workers, sit through a series of talks dealing with topics not usually discussed outside the female family circle. Relaxation exercises are seen as indecent and their purpose not readily associated with the Asian expectation of birth. An alternative system of parent education must be provided.

Organisation

The arrangement of parentcraft sessions for Asians is dependent upon a number of factors. These include the size and composition of the group, the location and timing of classes, and the availability of interpreters.

Numbers should be small enough to allow informality; twelve is about right but any accompanying female relatives should also be included as their influence on the mother-to-be is considerable and they will share in the upbringing of the baby. It is quite possible that relatives will outnumber mothers – this is all to the good.

The ideal group consists of women who share the same religion and mother tongue. It is preferable not to cater for all minorities together, although in a multi-ethnic area where numbers are small, this can be difficult to avoid. We have attempted to teach such groups and the results were chaotic. Our pearls of wisdom had to be translated simultaneously, into at least three different languages, with noise levels approaching those in the Tower of Babel. We suspect that we were less than effective.

Choosing a venue is not easy. Groups can fail because, despite careful organisation and sympathetic canvassing, the women were unable to make even a short journey outside their homes. The reasons can be found in earlier chapters. If link workers can act as an escort and are trusted by the mothers and their families, there might be an audience but only a few areas are blest in this respect. Workers must fall back on what we have found to be the only viable alternative which is to hold classes in conjunction with antenatal clinics. So much time is spent waiting for attention that it seems logical to offer health education to all mothers, regardless of their ethnic origins. Some hospitals have installed consumer operated videos and tape/slide presentations which can be of value to Asian mothers but should only be considered as supplementary to teacher-led groups.

The choice between hospital, health centre or surgery depends on the circumstances that prevail in each area. Hospitals have the best facilities but the most red tape, and mothers receiving antenatal care from a combination of hospital and general practitioner services may only visit a hospital clinic three times per pregnancy. G Ps can offer the best and the worst opportunities for parentcraft sessions. A well-motivated G P can organise her clinic to include time and facilities for teaching and give vital support in gaining the participation of mothers and their families. Surgery-based parentcraft allows the mother to develop a relationship with members of the Primary Health Care Team who will be looking after her and her baby. Locally-based midwives and health visitors can pitch their teaching to the known needs of their clients.

A health-centre-attached practice, while being less 'cosy', has the advantage of familiarising mothers with the local-authority-run child health services. There is usually access to health education resources.

Alas, the ideal is far removed from the reality that confronts many GP-attached health workers. We readily admit that apathy, indifference and even hostility may be met from colleagues, medical and otherwise, and that workers will have to muster their skills of perseverance and, in some instances, low cunning if they are to progress from pipedream to action. An example of the need for the last-mentioned skill comes from past experience of a practice, happily atypical, where co-operation was an unknown quantity. The only certainty in the fortnightly antenatal clinic was that the G P would be at least three-quarters of an hour late in arriving. By bringing all the appointment times forward there was enough time to carry out the routine observations and hold one, sometimes two, sessions of parentcraft before her arrival.

Interpreters are essential and should be a regular part of the teaching team. It is possible to 'make do' with an English-speaking mother from the group but this should be no more than a stopgap. Not only are the necessary skills likely to be absent but interpreting is a task few women relish. They dislike conveying messages that could cause offence and fear that they will become associated with the message and hence incur the disapproval of the group.

Topics

Having dealt with the organisational aspects of parenthood sessions, we can now turn to the content of these sessions, in which topics to be omitted are as important as those that are included.

Any subject covering anatomy or bodily functioning is best dealt with on a one-to-one basis. Intercourse during pregnancy, contraception and the physiology of labour are taboo for group discussion. Expressions of apprehension on the faces of the audience are more likely to be occasioned by the fear of embarrassment than the threat of labour pains, so it is worthwhile to explain at the outset that only 'safe' areas will be covered. In private, Asian women are prepared to talk about the most intimate matters, often questioning health workers with a frankness that is lacking in many native women.

We offer the following programme as a guideline only. So much depends on the women in the group and their needs that there can be no hard-and-fast rules.

Maintaining Health During Pregnancy

Most health educators like to devote their first session to this topic and, for obvious reasons, as early in pregnancy as possible. The major component is diet and if teaching is to be of any value, workers must have a detailed knowledge not only of traditional Asian eating patterns but also of the degree of adherence to those patterns. A parentcraft group could contain women who eat almost as they would in the subcontinent and, at the other end of the spectrum, women whose shopping baskets resemble those of their native neighbours. Differences are to be found within families where, for example, the newly-arrived bride might find that she is expected to tuck into fish and chips.

It is important to convince the audience that the teacher does know what she is talking about. Confidence rapidly drains away when it becomes evident that the advice offered stems from ignorance and false assumptions.

So what should pregnant Asian ladies eat and, more importantly, what do they eat?

The concept of food being eaten to maintain the body in balance was mentioned in Chapter 1 in connection with the Hindu lifestyle. Although Hindus attach the greatest significance to a correct balance between 'hot' and 'cold' foods, other Asians share the same philosophy to some extent, especially at times of illness or pregnancy. Confusingly, the categories of foods may vary between groups.

'Hot' and 'cold' foods as defined by Hindus

Hot	*Cold*
wheat	rice
potatoes	cows milk
buffalo milk	buttermilk
fish	green gram
chicken	chick peas
meat	peas
lentils	beans
ground nuts	onion
bitter gourd	green tomatoes
carrot	spinach
radish	brassicas
fenugreek	plantains
garlic	pumpkin
pawpaw	ripe mango
green mango	banana
dates	guava
eggs	lemon
	nuts

Some foods are omitted from these lists because they are regarded as neutral, conferring neither benefit nor harm. Apart from the fresh buffalo milk and some of the fruits, all the listed items are easily obtainable by the urban-dwelling British Asian, although at increased cost. Pregnancy is a 'hot' condition therefore 'hot' foods are avoided and 'cold' ones encouraged. The following nutritional advice should be relevant and acceptable to group members.

Protein The recommended daily intake of protein for pregnant women is 60g (Ministry of Agriculture, Fisheries and Food 1985). The following list shows the amount of food needed to yield 7g of protein:

1 oz meat	1 oz dried pulses (gram, dhal)
1 egg	1 oz nuts
$1\frac{1}{2}$ oz fish	3 oz cereals (flour, rice, chapatti)
$\frac{1}{3}$ pint of milk	1 oz cheese

(Spalding 1981)

Asian women derive much of their protein intake from dairy products and pulses. Meat-eating Moslems and Sikhs consume only small quantities, so where it is an accepted part of the diet meat should be recommended with other protein sources. Hard cheeses are not liked: they are unfamiliar and taboo because pigs' rennet is often used in their processing. Curd cheese can safely be recommended to all religious groups. Eggs are too 'hot' for Hindus but may be eaten by Moslems and Sikhs. Protein deficiency is considered to be one of the causes of intrauterine growth retardation (Dryburgh 1986) so if there are doubts about the adequacy of intake, supplementary protein should be recommended. One of the high protein meal replacement drinks should be acceptable because milk, which is drunk by most Asians, is used as a base but it should be stressed that it is to be taken in addition to normal meals.

Iron Pulses and green, leafy vegetables are the best sources of iron from the 'cold' list. An increased intake of vitamin C is advisable to aid the absorption of iron from vegetables. Iron supplements are usually taken as prescribed.

Folic Acid Fresh fruit and nuts should be eaten raw every day. As folic acid is destroyed by lengthy cooking, brassicas and pulses should only be lightly cooked. Supplementation in tablet form may be necessary.

Vitamin D Vitamin D deficiency does appear to affect Asians in Britain, the most likely reason being the paucity of sunlight available to synthesise the vitamin in dark-skinned people: Hindus seem to be the most disadvantaged in this respect (Shaunuk 1985). The recommendation that Asians should be screened and offered supplements if shown to be deficient, is not, at the time of writing, current practice.

Rickets can be acquired by the infants of severely vitamin D deficient women so advice is essential. Rickets was a problem in Britain in the early years of this century and was eventually overcome by the fortification of margarine, evaporated and infant formula milks, and the introduction of welfare vitamins. Margarine is not much used by Asians because some brands contain animal fats and traditionally, food is fried in clarified butter (ghee), although this is being replaced in popularity by vegetable oils. If ghee is used, it can be made with a mixture of half butter and margarine which can be recommended, together with brand names that do not violate religious laws. Evaporated milk can replace fresh milk when cocking sweets and puddings such as halva.

Clinics which sell baby milks also stock multivitamins, reasonably priced or free to pregnant women entitled to milk tokens. Multivitamins taken daily will ensure reasonable levels of all vitamins but women need to be warned that overdosages are harmful.

Calcium The intake of calcium is usually adequate because milk is a popular drink and is used in sweet cooking.

Fibre Constipation is one of the bugbears of pregnancy and workers expect to have to advise on ways of increasing fibre intake to offset the unfortunate effects of the action of progesterone on smooth muscle. As a nation, the British consumption of fibre is deplorably low, in marked contrast to those who adhere to an Asian diet. If members of the group are sufferers, the most likely cause is the abandonment of traditional eating patterns in favour of western foods.

Obesity and Gestational Diabetes Advice may be needed to prevent undesirably large weight gains and to reduce the risk of developing gestational diabetes, a condition which has a higher incidence among Asian women than is to be found in natives (Burden 1985). The message is the same for all would-be sensible eaters; to eat less fats, salts and sugars while maintaining consumption of foods essential for health. To be effective, one needs to know the calorie-laden culprits of the Asian diet. Drinks come high on the list of suspects. Tea, coffee and milk drinks are usually well sweetened, so conversion to artificial sweeteners could be of benefit. Soft drinks such as blackcurrant cordials and those high in glucose, often promoted as 'health products', are consumed in the mistaken belief that they are essential for health. Pure fruit juices are unsweetened and, therefore, a preferable alternative with some positive benefits to health.

Asian sweetmeats are death to the weight-conscious as the authors' expanding waistlines can testify. Do not forget to include British-style sweets, biscuits, crisps, cakes, and so on on the naughty list as they are becoming increasingly popular with Asian families. Before discouraging the consumption of fried foods, check whether the fat used is the only source of Vitamin D.

Fasting Fasting and diet are inseparable when considered in a religious context. Fasting has spiritual and health significance and is a feature of all three religions. Hindus moderate their fasts during pregnancy only by eschewing certain foods. Sikh women are less likely to fast than their Hindu sisters and when they do, a similar partial fast is observed.

The fast which worries many health workers is that carried out by Moslems during the month of Ramzan (Ramadan). Fasting is obligatory between the hours of sunrise and sunset with exemptions for menstruating, pregnant and lactating women who are expected to fast later in the year when their condition allows. Some devout Moslems fast despite their pregnancies and health workers have expressed concern at the possible harm to mother and child. Surprisingly, the reverse appears to be the case. A study of women in Birmingham showed that those women who adhered to the fast consumed the same or more in nutritional terms than those who ate normally (Eaton 1982). However, whether they fast or not, women find Ramzan a very tiring time. They are responsible for preparing the night-time meals which, if Ramzan falls in the summer months, entails going to sleep after midnight and rising before 4.00 am. Throughout the day normal household duties have to be performed and if there is a combination of toddlers and school children, opportunities for rest are minimal. This is when the audience of relatives can be encouraged to relieve the pregnant woman of some of her domestic burdens.

Alcohol, Smoking and Paan Native mothers expect to be warned of the dangers of smoking and alcohol taken during pregnancy. Only the most westernised of Asian women indulge openly in these particular 'vices' and they are not to be found in an Asian parentcraft class. We have come across a few smokers, mainly young British-educated girls, who smoke secretly in order not to incur family wrath. They would not admit publicly to their habit so anti-smoking advice to a class is less appropriate than in one-to-one counselling when smoking has been admitted. Some Asian women, notably from Bangladesh, chew Paan. Home visitors soon learn to recognise the small tray with its array of shiny leaves and pots of powders. Users have a characteristic red stain on their gums and teeth. The ingredients may vary according to region but among those commonly used are the leaves of the betel vine which has a carminative effect, to this is added the parings of areca nuts which are cholinergic and act as a stimulant, powdered lime, catechu which is a compressed extract from the uncaria gambia shrub, and finally, tobacco.

Women use Paan more than men. Indian women living in South Africa, who were studied by Schonland & Bradshaw (1969), claimed that when taken during the first trimester, Paan provides effective relief from nausea. In view of its contents and its known implication in upper alimentary canal cancer, health workers should advise caution. As yet, nothing is known about the effects on the fetus other than the acknowledged dangers of tobacco.

Breast Feeding

The promotion of breast feeding is as necessary for Asian mothers as it is for natives. Although breast feeding is the natural choice in the subcontinent, many women migrating in the sixties came at a time when artificial feeding was at the height of popularity, so they did as the natives. These women are now in a position to influence the current generation of young mothers and may try to persuade them that bottles are the smart, western way of feeding babies. Husbands have been exposed to advertising by the baby milk manufacturers and may also direct their wives towards the bottle. Families have a considerable 'say' in the choice between breast and bottle (Goel, House & Shanks 1978) so they should be included in any health education.

Care must be taken not to cause offence with terminology and illustration. The safest option is to refer to 'mother's milk'; diagrams of the process of lactation are best omitted as are slides, films and videos showing women breast feeding: in other words, stick to the benefits and leave out the mechanics. Mothers will appreciate being told that they may feed their babies in privacy while they are in hospital. Most have no objection to breast feeding in front of other women but will feel threatened by the male porters, doctors and relatives who visit the wards.

Attitudes to withholding colostrum can also be gauged and assurances given that wishes will be respected. Later, direct liaison with ward staff will ensure that mistakes are not made.

Diet during lactation can usefully be discussed. Mothers may alter their eating patterns to include 'hot' foods as a balance for the 'cold' condition of breast feeding, so advice must reflect this. The need to continue vitamin supplements should be stressed.

Artificial Feeding

There is some ambivalence in following a talk which promotes breast feeding with another teaching mothers how to prepare bottle feeds. However, whether by choice or circumstance, artificial feeding will be the method used by most mothers at some time, therefore it is essential that all should know how to prepare and give a feed using sterilised equipment.

We have found this a surprisingly difficult session to manage, needing meticulous interpreting and double-checking to make certain that the message has been accurately received. Health professionals dislike being authoritarian and aim to achieve change by reasoned persuasion, but our experience is that Asian women prefer a blunter approach and are not offended by imperatives. There is no place for euphemism when describing the consequences of incorrectly made feeds in unsterilised bottles: the baby will not be 'poorly', he will be very ill and could die.

A demonstration is obviously valuable but it may need to be repeated in the mother's home after the birth. It is difficult to discuss artificial feeding without appearing to promote a variety of products: choice may bewilder but is ethically more correct. This session provides an opportunity to tell mothers that SMA milks contain beef fat. Once a baby is established on SMA milk, the health worker has the unenviable choice between 'spilling the beans' which causes considerable distress, and keeping quiet in the hope that parents do not find out from some other source, risking an even greater upset if they do.

Many families live in houses with shared kitchens which do not have enough room to accommodate the paraphernalia needed for bottle feeding. Instead, everything is kept in the bedroom with boiled water stored in a thermos flask. There are dangers of infection attached to this practice and mothers should be warned in advance. Because artificial feeding is unfamiliar to so many women, the dangers of prop-feeding are also unknown and must be explained.

Baby Care in a Cold Climate

The aim is not to discourage patterns of infant care that are deeply rooted in Asian cultures, but to alert mothers to dangers that they have not previously encountered. Mothers do worry that their babies will catch cold and tend to go to the other extreme, overwrapping to such a degree that there is a risk of overheating. Advice should be included on when not to take the baby out of doors in bad weather.

What to buy in the way of equipment and clothing often causes anxiety, both financially and from a desire to 'do the right thing'. Baby clothes are of special interest as babies in the subcontinent wear very little, a cotton vest usually being sufficient. Manufacturers' catalogues are snapped up and invitations to accompany families on shopping trips are not unknown, although some prefer to delay the actual buying until the safe arrival of the baby, so as not to tempt fate. Nappies also deserve a mention. It is too hot for a baby to wear a nappy in many parts of the subcontinent instead, absorbent material is placed under the sleeping baby, and wrapped loosely around its middle at other times. In Britain, towelling nappies are being superseded in popularity by disposables, but enough parents still use them to justify a demonstration. Parents will then be able to make an informed choice between the two types of product.

Supermarket and chemist's shelves are filled to overflowing with wipes, oils, shampoos, bubble baths, ointments, creams and lotions, all marketed as essential for the well-cared-for baby and quite bewildering to the prospective Asian parents. A brief guide to what products are actually necessary and how these should be used will be welcome.

Washing powders and fabric softeners can irritate sensitive skins and advice can be given on the products that are best avoided.

What to Expect

Mothers appreciate knowing what to expect when they go into hospital and it is the 'hotel' aspects that are of greatest concern. Catering arrangements are probably top of the list, so the availability or otherwise of acceptable food can be outlined, as well as the attitudes of staff to food being brought in by relatives.

The list of articles to be brought into hospital on admission is another source of anxiety. Most Asians do not have separate night attire but sleep in clothing similar to that worn during the day. So long as whatever is worn does not obstruct nursing and medical care, most hospitals allow women to wear what they like.

Reassurance will also be appreciated that the need for privacy when praying will be respected, and that women confined to bed will be able to wash their hands beforehand.

Members of the group may have heard that it is the custom for fathers to be present during labour, and will be relieved that this is entirely optional and that a female friend or relative will be equally welcome. If the chosen lady speaks English her welcome will be even warmer as interpreters may not be available if the birth occurs 'out of hours'.

The roles of midwife, health visitor and general practitioner can be discussed, together with the services available at Child Health Clinics.

Finally, this is an excellent opportunity for encouraging the uptake of English as a Second Language and, if there are local schemes, *English for Pregnancy* tuition which, as was seen in Chapter 2, can be based in the home. If no such scheme exists and group members are keen to have one, the National Association for Teaching English as a Second Language to Adults might be willing to make provision.

The Father

Expectant Asian fathers are to be found at most antenatal clinics, waiting in an area apart from the women, as custom dictates. Their collective presence provides an ideal opportunity for preparing them for their role as a father in Britain.

The use of a female interpreter may cause offence and is not recommended. Most men have sufficient command of English to understand what is being said, and can interpret for the few non-speakers. As with their spouses, it is essential to start with assurances that neither family planning or anything remotely connected with their wives' anatomies will be discussed.

A new baby brings financial responsibilities. These can be outlined and advice given on how and where to claim appropriate benefits. The roles of midwife and health visitor should be included in the discussion, as should the services offered by the Child Health Clinics. If a husband has accompanied his wife to the antenatal clinic he will probably escort her to the baby clinic. The use of both facilities can be encouraged.

The advantages of English as a Second Language tuition can be added to this talk and information about local provision given. If nothing is available locally, husbands might consider teaching a few key phrases themselves, to ease the discomfiture of their wives' stay in hospital.

Information that health workers will be visiting the home after the birth can contain a plea for a stand-by interpreter who, it must be stressed, should be an adult and not a child kept home from school.

Men are not always aware of how tired their wives become towards the end of pregnancy and during the puerperium: the need for rest and a good diet should be stressed. Some help will be necessary if there are already young children in the family and if there is no available female support, the husband will have to take on some of the household and child care duties, which could be a new experience for him.

One of the benefits of this talk is an improvement in public relations. Asian men have varying impressions of female health professionals who, at best, are seen to be efficient but impersonal or, at worst, intolerant and prejudiced. Some suspect us of being proselytising feminists out to rock their matrimonial boats with our liberationist philosophy. If these fears can be dispelled the foundations will have been laid for an effective professional relationship.

Family Planning

Contraceptive advice is an integral part of health care and expectant parents are showered with information by professionals long before the baby is born. Workers are hesitant about broaching the subject with Asians for fear of causing offence, but this reticence does place couples at an unnecessary disadvantage.

Although attitudes to family planning vary between and within religions, family size does appear to be decreasing as lower infant mortality rates reduce the need for lots of babies in the hope that some will live to adulthood, and social conditions in Britain are not conducive to large families. However, the ideal size of an Asian family is larger than its native counterpart and health workers must make it clear that their aim is to help prevent unwanted pregnancies and not to interfere with desired family size.

Sikhs and Hindus, while endorsing the general view that children are a Divine blessing, do not appear unwilling to space their family or to prevent further pregnancies occurring when they feel their families are complete. There is confusion in the minds of health workers about Islamic teaching which, like Christian doctrine, is open to interpretation. The most orthodox Moslems refuse all contraception; others accept it provided that they can justify its use on health grounds because, as they see it, contraception is permissible only if the health of the woman is at risk should she become pregnant. This latter view seems to be held mainly by Bangladeshis. Some use contraception without any added justification but are anxious that no one else should know. A minority are uninhibited users.

Methods

The choice of method is determined by reliability, acceptability and the existence of possible side-effects. The oral contraceptive is widely known and usually accepted. In a young, non-smoking population the risk element is at its lowest. However, swallowing pills is a novel experience for most Asian women and it is essential that instructions are understood. Unless a domicilliary family planning service is available, women prefer to obtain their supplies from their general practitioners and not from the family planning clinics. This can result in less systematic follow-ups and poorer compliance rates. The unpleasant side-effects experienced during the first months' course should be explained, together with the need for extra protection.

Postnatal rubella screening and the offer of immunisation for those at risk gave rise to the need for foolproof contraception while the vaccine takes effect. Many women from the subcontinent had no immunity and were given the vaccine and an injection of Depo Provera at the same time. Not all of them were aware that one of the injections contained a contraceptive and they were extremely upset when enlightened. With other couples, Depo Provera proved popular with husbands because of the simplicity of administration and low failure rate, but less so with wives who disliked the disruption to their menstrual cycles and the weight gain that can be a side-effect. Since the drug has been licensed, our impression is that fewer women are being given it.

The intra-uterine contraceptive device is regarded with some suspicion. The fact that it is introduced vaginally deters a number of women, while its reputation for increasing menstrual bleeding is a minus point for women who are considered to be unclean during menstruation and barred from some domestic tasks. Women have also heard the same horror stories that frighten native women and are also suspicious that it is a form of sterilisation.

The diaphragm is not acceptable to the majority of Asian women because its insertion and removal offends against traditions of modesty, but as a method it should be included in any discussion on family planning so that the minority who might consider its use are made aware of its existence. Most men are prepared to use sheaths and some feel that control of fertility should be their responsibility anyway.

Cleverly marketed products such as foams, pessaries and creams may be purchased under the misapprehension that they are foolproof. Guidance is needed so that potential buyers only use them in conjunction with other methods.

Natural family planning is increasing in popularity as couples become disillusioned by the disadvantages of artificial methods. Asian couples might appear ideal candidates for this type of information but before offering a referral it is important to ascertain that teaching will not be carried out in a group setting.

Sterilisation is performed on both men and women in a minority of instances: few Asians are prepared to take such a drastic step. Abortion, too, is rarely carried out, being frowned upon, but not forbidden by all major faiths. If there is the likelihood of congenital malformation, some couples do accept termination, but they experience considerable guilt reactions and need sympathetic support.

We have found couples to be quite open about their views on family planning and have had no difficulty in gauging attitudes. It is important to appreciate that the extended family expect to have some influence on the couple and may like to be included in discussions. Inhibitions may creep in if an interpreter from their own community is present, with families unwilling to trust promises of confidentiality. A married woman of proven integrity is the ideal and on no account should an unmarried girl be used as an interpreter.

The best means of instruction is with the aid of a kit containing samples of the various methods. Information presented in this way is appreciated, and the worker can expect to be plied with a number of searching questions requiring explicit answers. Health education literature exists in abundance, much of it useless because of its over-reliance on the written word. If pictorial advice is given, the choice has to be made between the possibility of causing offence by the clarity of the message and creating confusion by ambiguity. Leaflets left in waiting rooms are likely to remain there as few Asians are willing to risk being seen reading them.

Communication aside, the main problem likely to be encountered is that of couples who disagree on family size, for example, the husband who disapproves of any intervention while his wife, worn out by frequent pregnancies, would give anything for some respite, and conversely, the devout wife who regards each pregnancy as a Gift of God while her husband appreciates the economic benefits of a small family. Showing respect for opposing views is difficult but nevertheless vital, as is support for the partner who 'loses'. Family friction can occur when couples are in agreement but go against the wishes of their elders.

The late Casper Brook (1981) believed that Family Planning Services lacked an essential ingredient – tender, loving care. We endorse the value of this often forgotten virtue and recommend its use in conjunction with technical expertise.

References

Black D (1982) In Davidson & Townsend (eds) *Inequalities in Health*. Harmondsworth: Pelican Books

Brook C (1981) *Family Planning for Immigrants – Report of a Symposium on the Health Needs of Ethnic Groups*. South Glamorgan Health Authority

Burden A (1985) Diet in gestational diabetes. *Practical Diabetes*, **2**(5), 15

Council for the Education and Training of Health Visitors (1977) *An Investigation into the Principles of Health Visiting*. London: CETHV

Dryburgh E (1986) Neonatal problems in the Asian population of Peterborough. *Midwife, Health Visitor & Community Nurse*, **22**, 1

Eaton P (1982) What do Asian women in Birmingham eat during pregnancy? *Proceedings of the Nutrition Society (London)*, **41**, 257

Goel, House & Shanks (1978) Infant feeding practices among Asians. *British Medical Journal*, 28 October

Hart J T (1971) The inverse care law. *Lancet*, **1**, 405–412

Ministry of Agriculture, Fisheries & Food (1985) *Manual of Nutrition*. London: HMSO

Schonland & Bradshaw (1969) Upper alimentary canal cancer in Natal Indians with special reference to the betel-chewing habit. *British Journal of Cancer*, **23**, 670–682

Shaunak S, Colston K, Ang L, Patel P & Maxwell J (1985) Vitamin D deficiency in adult British Hindu Asians: a family disorder. *British Medical Journal*, **291**, 1166–1168

Sibert J, Jadhavi M & Inbaraj S (1979) Fetal growth and parental consanguinity. *Archives of Disease in Childhood*, **54**(4), 317

Spalding D (1981) *The Nutritional Needs of Asian Immigrants – Report of a Symposium on the Health Needs of Ethnic Groups*. South Glamorgan Health Authority

Watson E (1984) Health of infants and use of services by mothers of different ethnic groups in East London. *Community Medicine*, **6**, 127–135

Wharton B (1982) *Topics in Perinatal Medicine*. London: Pitman Medical

Recommended Reading

Mares P, Henley A & Baxter C (1985) *Health Care in Multiracial Britain*. Cambridge: National Extension College/Health Education Council. Demonstrates the gaps in current health care for minority groups and aims to raise the general awareness of health workers; useful sections on family planning and haemoglobinopathies.

Chapter 4

INFANCY

The return home from hospital after childbirth forms one of the personal landmarks that remains forever in the memories stored by every woman who is a mother. She can recall the mixture of joy and apprehension, the optimism mingled with doubt about her ability to cope with the immense task ahead. These feelings are universal, part of the bond of experience that unites mothers irrespective of their race, creed, class or age. Asian mothers are as much a part of this sorority as any other group of women, but those who have borne and reared their children in Britain share an additional set of experiences which are unique and which neither native women nor those remaining in the subcontinent can fully understand. For these ladies, life is a balancing act in which the traditional child-rearing practices of the Asian family have to be weighed against the practical considerations of life in northern Europe and the alien but 'expert' advice of health professionals. Into this equation enters the mother's own perceptions and expectations which complete a triangle of stress and conflict in which she attempts to compromise between widely differing means to the common end of a successfully reared child.

Under ideal circumstances there should be no conflict; health workers would have a sound knowledge of Asian cultures and would be free from ignorance and prejudice, treating with respect the manifestly positive aspects of traditional customs and seeking only to adapt and not to suppress practices which are incompatible with life in Britain. Support from interpreters and ESL provision would enable two-way communication between client and worker who would already have achieved common ground through the medium of culturally acceptable preparation for parenthood classes.

Sadly, the reality is less than perfect: the Health Service has yet to adopt a multicultural approach, leaving its workers bereft of resources and its Asian clientele with such a depth of suspicion that good care is in danger of being rejected along with the bad.

The purpose of this chapter is to translate the child care expertise that is part of the health worker's repertoire into a realistic and culturally acceptable resource with which to guide Asian families through the early stages of childhood.

Naming The Baby

One of the first questions asked of new parents is 'What is the baby's name?' Most native parents decide on forenames well in advance of the birth and it is unusual for a baby to remain unnamed for more than the first few days of life. Names are chosen by the parents with only scant deference being paid to the views of the extended family. Asian families follow different customs based on their religious beliefs which, unless they are understood by health workers, can lead to confusion and misinformation being fed into computers.

Most Moslem couples ask the paternal grandparents to choose the name and if they are living in the subcontinent several weeks may elapse before the choice is made known to the parents in Britain. All the grandchildren's names share a common theme; they might commence with the same initial or be part of a rhyming scheme, or perhaps the girls are named after flowers. As the given name comprises two or three elements, possibly all different from those of the parents, we again endorse Alix Henley's advice (1979) to record the full name, underlining the personal name and adding the father's final name: eg. Mohamed *Asim,* son of Tariq *Iqbal,* or *Fatima* Bibi, daughter of Tariq *Iqbal.* The records for all members of the family should then be filed under the name 'Iqbal'.

Hindu naming customs vary according to region and degree of westernisation. One with which we have become familiar entails the date and hour of birth being submitted to a priest who casts the baby's horoscope, the result of which determines the initial letter of the name. The joint family then confer and decide on the full name which will also form part of a pattern for all the children of the family.

Sikhs, too, vary in their naming customs but those following the orthodox tradition have a special naming ceremony, when the family and friends gather together and after prayers have been said, the Holy book, the Guru Granth Sahib, is opened at random and the initial letter of the first word on the page is to be the first letter of the child's name. The full name, which can be used for boys or girls, is then chosen by the family.

Parents must obtain a birth certificate from the Registry office within six weeks of the birth. This is usually time enough for a name to have been given but, in the event of delays, Registrars are willing to extend the time limit as any subsequent alteration entails lengthy and expensive paperwork.

If the Registry Office allows for flexibility, the health authority computer does not. Even as the baby is being discharged from hospital the computer is busy digesting the mother's name for use as a surname, with the result that records are sent to the health visitor for a male baby Begum, Kaur or Bibi. Any incorrect data is usually amended on the form consenting to immunisation appointments which is signed by parents at the primary birth visit and subsequently fed into the computer. This is still too soon for most Asian babies to have been named so when the family keep their first immunisation appointment confusion is inevitable because the baby has acquired a name which does not tally with that on the printout. The only way around this is to ensure that the father's name is on the consent form and that parents are told that appointments will be addressed to 'the parents of . . . (father's name)'. At the first immunisation the correct name can be given with special attention being paid to the spelling which can vary because it is a translation of a different script but it does need to be constant for record keeping. The father's name should be retained as the key family surname. Ideally, computers should be programmed to accept Asian naming systems, thereby reducing the likelihood of errors.

Once the baby has been named one might assume that the health worker's difficulties are at an end but there are still pitfalls for the unwary. Like the natives, Asian parents use nicknames and terms of endearment so perhaps the baby who does not respond to his name when hearing is being assessed has never heard it used. More than one baby in the early days of our practice has been recorded as the Asian equivalent of 'darling' – Patel, Kaur or Miah.

Boys Better Than Girls?

The desire for sons is often misunderstood as disappointment at the birth of a daughter. This is rarely the case, as seasoned health workers will have already observed. Sons are important: in an agrarian society sons are needed to work the land, and for Hindus it is the son who performs the funeral rites. Asians come from a patrilocal society where we find the converse to the old adage 'Your son is your son till he gets him a wife, and your daughter's your daughter for all of her life'. Although the giving of a dowry is officially discouraged, in the subcontinent as in many other countries, it is a custom that dies hard and parents expect to go to some expense when the daughters are of marriageable age. Rearing a daughter in Britain with its apparent endorsement of sexual freedom, is a prospect which worries most Asian parents, who would probably agree that daughters are more of a responsibility than sons. However, parents with a number of sons are as likely to long for a daughter as are their native neighbours. A daughter promises help for the hard-pressed mother as well as much needed female company, nevertheless it is a reasonable assumption that parents without sons will probably keep 'trying' until they produce one. A referral to the Roman Catholic Natural Family Planning Association could prove productive as they also advise on the timing of intercourse to increase the chances of conceiving a baby of the desired sex. One family with a clutch of daughters was more than delighted when the counselling received resulted in the birth of twins, yet another girl and the longed-for son.

Infant feeding looms large among the topics brought to the health worker for advice, and only a tiny minority of babies sail through the months of milk feeds and weaning diets without a few hiccups and allied aberrations. The baby is not the least concerned about the traditional feeding customs of his mother but may voice his objections if she is tense and anxious because she has been subjected to a plethora of conflicting advice and does not know which to follow. We have considered breast and bottle feeding as part of the preparation for parenthood – how can the mother be helped to turn theory into practice?

Breast Feeding

The numbers of Asian mothers leaving hospital with fully-breast-fed babies are disappointingly low and they become even fewer after a few weeks at home. The disincentives to breast feed have already been discussed but why should the mother who has opted for this method of feeding fail in her declared aim?

One potent reason is almost certainly the inability to communicate with those in a position to help, both in hospital and at home. Advice and encouragement from professionals and self help groups such as the National Childbirth Trust and the Association of Breast feeding Mothers can make all the difference to the unconfident new mother, offering support through the early days of engorgement, sore nipples and failed let-down reflexes. The basis of this support is verbal interaction; mother expresses her worries, the counsellor advises on a change of tactics or encourages perseverence. Non-English-speaking mothers are denied this help, except in areas well supplied with interpreters, and for the most part, struggle on unaided.

In the subcontinent, because there is a defined lying-in period during which the mother cares only for her baby, she is able to offer the baby feeds on demand without the stress of other domestic commitments. Although native mothers no longer feed by the clock, they do have to cope with housework, shopping, cooking, and so on, and expect a reasonable breather between feeds. The Asian mother living in Britain must perforce follow a similar pattern, but with the added knowledge that this is not the way she would have followed in her country of origin.

Confidence in her ability to breast feed successfully is further sapped if the new mother is unable to adapt her eating pattern to accommodate those foods which are believed to promote lactation. She wants to eat 'hot' foods to counteract her 'cold' condition but may have difficulty in obtaining them and insufficient time in which to cook separately for herself.

Breast feeding is not an activity to be carried out in the presence of men. Although clothing can be arranged so that the baby feeds easily and discreetly, there is unease if men are in the same room. Not all British homes are big enough to provide separate quarters for men and women so in order to obtain the necessary privacy, the mother may have to leave the living room and retreat to her bedroom every time the baby wants to feed.

If the Hindu or Sikh mother has chosen not to suckle the baby before her milk 'comes in', establishing lactation may take some time and without help can be difficult to accomplish, especially if formula milks have been given in the meantime. On the other hand, if the girl has been persuaded to feed from the start, she could be feeling anxious about the possible harm done to her baby by the violation of a cultural practice in which she sincerely believes.

Because there is a tendency for Asian babies to be 'light for dates' professionals are keen to maximise 'catch-up' growth and may misguidedly suggest complementary feeding which will probably result in understimulation of lactation and, ultimately, failure of supply. Other workers, uncertain of the mother's nutritional state and anxious to prevent vitamin deficiencies, may also recommend formula milks.

Pressure from members of the family with experience only of artificial feeding may further dent the resolve of the new mother. It is worth remembering that it is the family-in-law with whom the new mother is living and not her own family; thus, if pregnancy occurred soon after the marriage she may still be settling into her new home and developing a relationship with her in-laws which she would not wish to prejudice by ignoring their advice.

Finally, a number of Hindu and Sikh women take maternity leave from their employment and plan to return to work soon after the birth. They may not realise that it is possible to continue breast feeding even though mother and child are apart during the day.

In summation, those most likely to breast feed their babies for months rather than weeks are the women who are well-integrated into their extended families and where the women of those households have experience of and are committed to breast feeding. Such a mother will have had her wishes regarding colostrum understood and respected by postnatal ward staff and will have access to interpreters so that she may ask for and receive advice. Her home circumstances will be such that she has privacy from men and enough female help to enable her to enjoy a lying-in similar to that in the subcontinent. Her professional advisers will be well versed in Asian child-rearing practices.

What can the health worker do to help those who probably form the majority of Asian women in Britain and have few of the aforementioned advantages? Admittedly, not a great deal; she cannot alter the geography of the mother's home, neither can she remove all the domestic pressures that afflict the modern woman. She is also at the mercy of her employing authority as to whether the communications hurdle can be overcome. She can ensure that members of the primary health care team are made aware of the value of breast feeding and even when differences of opinion are expressed, she can state her commitment, leaving colleagues in no doubt as to how she advises her mothers. She can encourage the intake of foods that are culturally acceptable and maintain health; lentils, in particular, are considered to be beneficial to the lactating mother and are a good source of protein. Dairy products are also eaten and although on the 'cold' list, milk is drunk provided it has been warmed. Advice can be given to the woman who has to eat the normal family diet, on which foods such as garlic and hot spices should be avoided because they could upset the baby. Multivitamins and iron supplements will boost maternal nutrition. Aids which help to overcome some of the early problems of breast feeding such as topical pain relief, nipple shields and breast pumps can be demonstrated. Worries that the baby is not thriving on breast milk should be dispelled by weighing the baby, at home if possible, so that sceptical relatives can see for themselves that this method of feeding does have merits.

The impact of this piecemeal approach will inevitably be limited and if the promotion of breast feeding is to achieve positive results we need to rethink our policies. We believe that there is a place for breast feeding counsellors, trained to promote and sustain breast feeding among the Asian population. Ideally, the counsellor should have a similar cultural background to her clients and should be married with personal experience of breast feeding. A nursing background would be a bonus but communication skills are more important. Training could come from one of a number of agencies, including the National Childbirth Trust who have already demonstrated their desire to be multicultural in their appeal by producing health education leaflets in the main Asian languages. The counsellor's role during the antenatal period, would include promotion of breast feeding perhaps participating in some of the parent-craft sessions outlined in the previous chapter. After delivery, the counsellor would visit mothers in hospital and later, at home. Part of her role would be to educate the professionals and to liaise with those working with the mother in the community. The cost of such counsellors should be more than offset by the reduction in expensive hospital admissions for artificially-fed babies suffering from gastroenteritis.

The accusation that special provision for Asian mothers is yet one more act of racism on the part of the health service can be countered by arguing that the current provision is in itself racist as only those subscribing to western cultural values benefit from it. We should also remember that those Asian mothers who want to breast feed experience the same feelings of failure as natives when they do not succeed. The yardstick for measuring the success of any extension to the service should include a large measure of consumer satisfaction.

Artificial Feeding

The bottle-fed Asian baby has become the norm. If women have chosen not to breast feed it is essential that formula milk feeds should be accurately prepared and given with the minimum risk of infection. Jivani (1978) observed that hospital admissions were higher for the bottle-fed babies of immigrants than they were for native babies.

The mother who has attended parentcraft classes has a head start and she is also likely to receive a further demonstration of feed-making techniques during her stay on the postnatal ward. Mothers, overwhelmed by the excitement of the birth, are not always at their most receptive at this time and, unless an interpreter is present, a demonstration without any verbal explanation could confuse rather than clarify. There is a case for repeating the demonstration of making up feeds and bottle sterilisation once mother and baby have returned home. Teaching can then be adapted to suit domestic circumstances.

We have found that most parents use a cold water steriliser, usually a purpose-made unit. Although these are expensive, when communication is difficult, it is easier to demonstrate the need for exact quantities of water because there is a permanently-marked water line. Our experience is that parents do appreciate the importance of scrupulous attention to hygiene but that there are areas of confusion; for example, the need to rinse sterilising fluid out of the bottle with boiled water; another is ensuring that the water used to make the feed is at the correct temperature. We have already mentioned the dangers associated with vacuum (Thermos) flasks used to store off-the-boil water overnight. Another potential source of infection is the half-finished bottle which may be kept in case the baby wants an in-between-feeds snack. This ties in with the Asian practice of frequent demand feeding which can result in the bottle being constantly available, which does pose a serious health risk. Other than keeping a supply of prepared bottles in the 'fridge', there is no alternative to making a fresh feed every time the baby is hungry.

The custom of breast feeding the baby for longer than is usual with natives is carried over to bottle feeding. Weaning on to a cup before the first birthday is very uncommon and it is considered appropriate for drinks to be given via a bottle until the child is three or even older, with disastrous effects on dental health when sweetened drinks are given. Once it has been appreciated that sugary drinks sucked from a bottle are harmful, parents try to break what has become an entrenched habit, often with great difficulty. Discouraging the use of baby juices until they can be drunk from a cup may prevent the habit from being formed, as will the gradual introduction of a cup from the age of six to nine months. The occasional 'comfort' bottle of unsweetened milk is not likely to harm the older toddler and should not be discouraged as this may be seen as a criticism of cultural practices.

Formula milks are expensive and time-consuming in their preparation so it is hardly surprising that parents are keen to change over to 'doorstep' milk at the earliest opportunity. Unfortunately, the early introduction of whole cows' milk means that the baby may become deficient in the extra vitamins and iron that are added to formula milks. He may also be unable to cope with the increased solute load. Black (1985) recommends that Asian babies should remain on formula milks until they are one year old, and in line with D H S S recommendations advises the use of vitamin drops between the ages of one month and five years. Advice to parents not to wean on to 'doorstep' milk should begin well before the baby is six months old otherwise the message might come too late. A reminder should be given not to add sugar or rusk to the bottle: milk is not usually drunk unsweetened by Asians but change is necessary if children are to be spared hours of dental treatment.

Another source of sugar much enjoyed by the baby is gripe-water. Few health workers actually recommend the use of these products as they are over sweet and their effectiveness against colic has yet to be proven. However, they are popular with mothers and we have noticed that the dosage instructions are followed meticulously, irrespective of any perceived need. The health visitor will of course, have all the answers to colic problems!

Weaning

When and how to give the baby solid food has probably caused health visitors more grey hairs than any other health care issue. Britain has seen a number of changes in weaning policy and our credibility with the public has suffered as a result. The 'sixties saw us persuading mothers to offer their babies solids from the age of four weeks and giving those whose infants tucked into beef broth, chicken and veg, and so on, an extra pat on the back. During the 'seventies there was a complete reversal for this school of thought, when the dangers of over-loaded kidneys and hypernatraemia became evident – nothing but milk until the baby was four months old. Hungry babies and their protesting mothers have brought about a modification and three months is now reckoned to be a safe time to begin weaning. As the problems associated with the early consumption of wheat are now recognised, gluten-free products are recommended for the young weanling. Salt and sugar are also taboo, while increasing concern is being focused on food additives – home cooking is encouraged but can we be certain that some of the ingredients used are not harmful?

Against this background of continuously emerging knowledge the health worker has to advise mothers from all ethnic origins, and it is hardly surprising that she finds difficulty in getting across such a complicated aspect of health education to those with little command of English and very different traditions of infant feeding. Babies are not given solids in the subcontinent until they are at least a year old, then they are fed the cereal that predominates in their region. Gujaratis mix rice and dhal into a kedgeree, Punjabis give softened chapatis and Bangladeshis make a rice gruel. From this the young child graduates to family food, although it may be some years before hotly spiced foods are enjoyed. Madhur Jaffrey, the actress and writer of cookery books, recalls that her liking for adult food was not fully developed until she was nine years old.

The advice given to native mothers wishing to wean their babies is simply inappropriate for Asian families, who are being asked to change not only the contents of weaning foods but also the timing of their introduction. The role of the health worker is to ensure that the family understands the need for an earlier introduction and to suggest those foods that are compatible with traditional patterns. Black (1985) and Ehrhardt (1986) point to the dangers of iron deficiency anaemia if a milk-only diet is followed and there is evidence that low serum iron concentrations are associated with an increased susceptibility to infection Bondestam (1985). This appears to justify the commencement of solids at not later than six months when fetal iron stores have become depleted.

Asian mothers are willing to give early solids but need more guidance than native mothers because of the difficulty of finding suitable foods. The standard introductory rice-based cereal is always acceptable. Here, sample packets have their uses because the worker can read through the list of contents with family members to reassure them that it conforms with religious beliefs. Different proprietory brands should always be mentioned so as not to bias choice. There is no reason why mothers should not make their own rice cereal and those keen to do so should be encouraged, but at the same time, advised not to use 'doorstep' milk or too much sugar and only to use a small amount of water to clean the rice, thus retaining as much of the water-soluble B vitamins as possible.

That was the easy part. Native mothers are next advised to give a little pureed vegetable as a second meal in order to cultivate a liking for savoury foods, as most health workers have accepted the current view that too much sweet food early in life is responsible for all sorts of ills later on. Asian weaning foods are invariably sweet and the recipes quoted by Jivani

(1978) which are nutritionally sound and based on protein foods such as lentils (dhals), ground nuts and millets, are sweetened with jaggery, also known as gur, an unrefined palm sugar, rich in iron. Jaggery is available in Britain but is approximately three times the price of granulated sugar which may be used as a substitute. The use of refined sugars should be actively discouraged, but we think it preferable to accept the sweetening of vegetables with raw sugars as part of a rich culinary heritage, the abandonment of which could lead to the adoption of some of the less desirable aspects of western diet.

While nothing in a tin or packet can compare with home cooking using freshly acquired ingredients, all mothers would agree that the non-availability of convenience baby foods would increase their workload and make life far less easy. If it is wrong to deny the benefits of instant baby food to native mothers it is equally wrong so to deprive Asian mothers. In the past few years manufacturers have woken up to the fact that not everyone is carnivorous and the subsequent growth in vegetarian baby foods has been a boon for the Asian family. There are snags; health workers need to become compulsive packet readers to ensure that what they recommend does not have any hidden extras. One manufacturer of dehydrated baby foods adds meat extract to over half its vegetable varieties, making them unsuitable for all religious groups. Another company has only recently changed its feeding advice literature which had previously illustrated a sareed lady opening a tin of chicken dinner, a picture likely to offend Moslems and Hindus. Consumer mistrust is wholly understandable and it is another reason for cupboards being stocked with tins of egg custard and other sweet varieties.

As the baby approaches his first birthday, his mother may be advised to give him family foods without the spices. This is to misunderstand the nature of Asian cookery where spices are the first ingredients to be cooked, the meat, poultry or vegetables then being fried in the spice-impregnated oil. It is more realistic to suggest that the morsels for the baby be cooked as usual but without additional salt, and then rinsed to remove the traces of hot spices. Foods cooked in mild spices such as cardamom, cummin and coriander can be eaten quite safely by the older baby, and it is advisable that these be given in infancy as there is a danger that the toddler fed exclusively on bland food may reject family foods when they are eventually offered.

So far, advice has been aimed at the client who wishes to follow traditional weaning patterns and to conform with religious dietary doctrines; not all Asian families fall into this category so workers must gauge attitudes before they offer guidance. The majority of Moslems do not want their offspring to eat any meat that is not Halal although a few may accept meat that has been through British slaughterhouses, avoiding only pork: thus, most manufactured baby foods are acceptable to a minority. Vegetarian Sikhs and Hindus may wish to give their children meat during their growing years, and boys especially, are encouraged to eat chicken and lamb. Others prefer to give foods from vegetable sources only.

Some women may have evolved a lifestyle far removed from that of their parents and grandparents, with religious affiliations being mainly nominal, and they could be genuinely offended by the health workers assumptions that their offspring are to be fed in accordance with the Asian traditions that they have eschewed. The response of these ladies should not be confused with that of the mother who, sensing the health worker's disapproval of Asian feeding practices, appears to accept advice on native foods which, if acted upon, would compromise her beliefs and cherished values. Both examples could have been avoided if the mother had been able to express her views to a worker whom she trusted not to impose her own value judgements.

Audiotapes are ideal for the transmission of weaning advice to the non-English-speaker and can be accompanied by pictures of the foods included in the script. Appendix 1 offers specimen scripts which can be adapted to suit specific needs.

Growth Patterns

The birth weight of the average Asian baby is lower than that of his native counterpart but, as de Lobo (1978) points out, this need not cause undue alarm unless there is evidence that the baby has suffered from intra-uterine growth retardation (IUGR); often babies are of low birth weight because they have been born to parents of short stature and are themselves small. In view of the hazards of hypoglycaemia, poor temperature control and infection to which the IUGR baby may succumb in the immediate postnatal period, the early identification of those at risk is essential. Centile charts have proved invaluable in monitoring the health of native babies but, according to Meadows (1986), they tend to give an overestimation of IUGR when applied to Asian babies. A more accurate prediction can be obtained by measuring the ratio of mid-arm circumference to occipitofrontal circumference, the ratio remaining constant for healthy infants irrespective of their ethnic origins and their position on the centile chart, but showing a deviation in those infants with IUGR who subsequently develop symptoms. Mid-arm circumference to occipitofrontal circumference ratios may be used to gauge the progress of older Asian babies for whom weight charts standardised on native babies may be inappropriate.

Asian parents are often worried about the physical development of their children and require frequent reassurance that growth rates are within normal limits and that the baby is healthy. Hindu and Sikh mothers may monitor their babies' growth themselves and workers will sometimes observe a thin strip of elasticated material tied around the wrist with, perhaps another around the midriff. As the baby gains weight the slack in the band is taken up, giving the mother positive feedback. Some women also believe that the presence of the bands actually promotes growth so they do have an additional 'talisman' effect. A tiny scroll in a metal case may be attached which has religious significance.

Because there is such anxiety about growth, the baby who gains weight rapidly and hits the 90th centile is a source of great pride to his parents. Obesity is a sign of wealth, indicative of a father able to provide more than enough for his family's needs. Seen against a background of subsistence farming with the threat of famine ever present, this attitude is more than understandable and very difficult to change, particularly as the Asian practice of frequent demand feeding, perfectly designed for the small baby, is also to the liking of the greedy whopper who has only to open his mouth for his 'hunger' to be instantly gratified.

Immunisation

Immunisation is readily accepted by Asian parents who may have had first-hand experience of the devastation caused by infectious diseases. Although figures are not available for the rate of uptake, we suspect that in South Glamorgan they are certainly as high, if not higher, than those for natives.

The problems that do arise are mainly those of communication. Few doctors are happy to immunise a baby unless they can be sure that the child is in good health, has no adverse neonatal or family history, and that the current immunisation status is known. They also like to advise parents on aftercare and the recognition of side effects. This essential information cannot be transmitted if the parent's command of English is poor and if there is no interpreter. GP-run immunising clinics offer some advantages over child health clinics; the patients are known to the immunising doctors and medical records can readily be consulted. If the baby is to be immunised at a child health clinic by a clinical medical officer who may not know the family or have access to an interpreter, the role of the health visitor is crucial. She can warn parents when and where appointments are due and suggest that an English-speaker accompanies the mother. She can ensure that any contraindications are written on the record kept by the family and on that held by the clinic.

The only difference in the immunisation programme is that Asian babies are more likely to be offered protection against tuberculosis. As there is an increased susceptibility to TB among the Asian population (Campbell 1981), it makes sense to protect children at the earliest opportunity from what is still a lengthy and debilitating illness. If the baby is less than six weeks old BCG vaccine can be given without prior skin testing. Although Grindulis (1984) found that 50% of babies who had received BCG were negative to Mantoux testing at 22 months, Hadfield (1986) claims a post-BCG immunity of 75% for both babies and adolescents provided vaccinations are given by experienced workers using the Dermojet method.

The circumstances in which the vaccine is given depends on area policy: some babies are vaccinated before leaving hospital which seems to us to be the ideal; in other areas, our own included, appointments are offered to all babies with Asian surnames. The attendance rate in South Glamorgan is excellent despite the difficulties encountered by parents who have to attend one of only three clinics offering BCG in the county. Hindu and Sikh mothers who traditionally do not leave their homes for six weeks post-delivery, invariably find someone to take the baby. This system is preferable to differing provision being available within the same authority where, for example, one hospital routinely offers BCG vaccination to Asian neonates while parents of babies delivered in the hospital down the road, have to make their own arrangements. We do think there should be a nationwide standardisation in the provision of BCG vaccination.

Developmental Screening Tests

All parents are offered screening tests to check that their offspring's development is progressing normally. Some are carried out by the health visitor, either in the home or at the child health clinic, and others are performed by clinical medical offers. A small but increasing number are screened by their G P. Verbal interaction between parent and tester is essential if an accurate assessment is to be accomplished and clinical medical officers may experience difficulties similar to those described in the section on immunisation, in that they are unlikely to know the family and have only the barest of details, on the clinic record card. Developmental progress such as the age at which the baby first smiled or sat unsupported, can only be ascertained by asking the parent. Without a common language, developmental screening represents a poor return on expensive manpower for the NHS and can only be a threatening and bewildering experience for parents, doing little to encourage the further uptake of services.

Confusion can arise because Asian parents may calculate their baby's age differently from natives. For instance, a native mother identifies her baby as being six months old after it has completed its sixth month of life, some Asian parents might describe their baby as being six months old once the fifth month has passed. This presents no problem when the baby's current developmental status is being assessed but it could give a false impression of a delay if, for example, the mother recalls the age at which the baby first smiled as being two months which would be abnormally late, although by native reckoning the baby was only one month old and well within the normal range.

Difficulties may be encountered when administering to Asians screening tests which have been standardised on children reared in western culture. A number of health authorities use the Denver Developmental Screening practices, in particular those assessing the child's personal/social development. As we have shown, babies rarely drink from a cup before the age of one so they are unlikely to have aquired sufficient skill in manipulating a cup without spilling the contents to score a pass by the 16-month deadline. Many families prefer to use the right hand instead of cutlery for eating which nullifies the item on the ability to manage a spoon. Similarly, independence as measured by the child being able to dress himself is not so highly valued as it is in native families so much of this section will be invalidated by the number of 'no opportunity' responses. The motor section presents few problems as it is the child's actions that are being tested and our impressions are that Asian babies score slightly higher than natives. Assessing language development presents a number of problems especially when dealing with the older baby; an accurate result is impossible without an interpreter if the parent does not have a complete command of English. Children are usually brought up to speak the mother tongue, perhaps picking up a little English if there are older school children living in the household. Parents may not understand that when assessing language development workers are not concerned which language is spoken: we have been assured by parents that children are unable to speak at all when they are fluent in their own language. A health worker with a knowledge of Asian languages is at an advantage when testing items which require worker/child interaction such as picture recognition and the identification of parts of the body. Armed with a small vocabulary (see Appendix 2) the worker can enjoy a direct relationship with the child, enhancing her own pleasure and can, by listening to the child's response, be absolutely sure that the item has been achieved. Until we learnt that 'billee' is Punjabi for 'cat' we were unaware of the amount of maternal prompting that took place.

Safety

Parents are always anxious to protect their offspring from accidental injury. Those with an imperfect command of English may feel especially vulnerable when confronted with unfamiliar equipment and product instructions which are incomprehensible. Time spent by the health worker explaining potential dangers is usually appreciated and the advice given is invariably followed.

Pillows have long been a bone of contention between health worker and mother and we suspect that many a woman, irrespective of her ethnic origins, does a vanishing act with the forbidden article at the approach of the health visitor. Asian mothers like using pillows but are willing to discontinue their use once the danger is made known. Some mothers place a pad of fabric under the baby's head and the dangers here are that any loose materials could block the airway, and should vomiting occur drainage may be impeded by lack of absorbency or by the position of the material close to the nose and mouth.

Baby nests have become very popular items of equipment and are used by Asians probably as a cosy antidote to the British climate. Following catastrophes in which the inner quilting caused suffocation, the manufacturers changed the type of fabric and attached a warning label to the effect that babies should not use the nests for sleeping unless they can be closely and continuously observed. It is this last point that needs to be emphasised especially as the nest may appear to be the ideal container for the baby who sleeps in the maternal bed. Prop-feeding has already been mentioned (see Chapter 3), but not all members of the family may have received the message, so reinforcement is advisable.

Asian babies are not separated from the rest of the household and are usually left to sleep amidst the activity of the living area. Sometimes a pram is used but more often the baby is placed on the settee and this has its dangers if there are small children about or if the baby has reached the rolling-over stage. In a family with plenty of adults, one of whom is always watching over the children, this practice presents few hazards but most women have to fit in household chores which prevents complete attention being focused on the baby, so workers should recommend a less precarious resting place.

Advice about animals and their health hazards is not usually necessary because not many Asian families have household pets. However, if the family have a garden in which to put the pram, they need to know about protective netting against the neighbours' cats and everybody's insects. Putting the baby out into the fresh air is not common practice in the subcontinent for obvious reasons, but it is worth encouraging in Britain if only for the additional vitamin D gained, the exceptions being those living in the inner cities where the benefits may be offset by the adverse effects of atmospheric pollution.

As the baby becomes mobile so the risk of accidents increases. Safety gates and fireguards are immediately procured once the need is made known. Playpens are not popular; the idea of placing a baby inside a cage filled with toys does not tally with the Asian concept of parenting. On the other hand, baby walkers are used and accidents have occurred because their dangers have not been appreciated. Steps between rooms are a feature of the older type of house often occupied by city-dwelling families and these have contributed to a number of nasty injuries involving walkers.

An urban environment is a good deal more hostile a place in which to play than a rural village in the subcontinent. A typical parental reaction is a strong desire to keep everyone indoors so as to avoid the dangers outside. Less common, is a failure to appreciate the risks and allow very young toddlers to play in the street in the charge of their not much older siblings. Little children, especially girls, do handle babies rather more than their native peers, both in and out of doors. There can be few more heart-stopping sights than that of a five-year-old struggling to negotiate the stairs with a boisterous one-year-old in her arms. Stairs are not usually a feature of housing in the subcontinent, indeed, 'bungalow' is a Hindi word and describes exactly the accommodation migrating families have left behind them. The dangers attached to two-storey living need to be explained.

Parents may be unaware of the legal consequences of leaving young children unattended and that should an accident occur when children under the age of sixteen are unsupervised in the home, they are liable to prosecution, a fact which surprises a number of native parents and is greeted with disbelief by Asians who expect teenaged children to manage their young siblings with competency. Making safe arrangements for the care of children when mother has to 'pop out' for a few minutes, has been a problem experienced by only a small minority of women prior to their arrival in Britain, the joint family ensuring that someone is always available to care for them. Mothers in Britain, irrespective of their ethnic origins, face enormous difficulties in coping with small children when shopping or collecting older children from school; cleaning and dressing up against the vagaries of the climate, crossing roads against traffic which makes no allowance for walkers proceeding at toddler pace, heaving a pram up and down kerbsides with only one hand because the other one has tight hold of a toddler with Houdini tendencies; small wonder a few succumb to the temptation to trust to luck that the baby will stay asleep in his cot for the short while that mother is away. The only difference between Asian and native mothers is that the native has been conditioned not to leave her child unattended and takes a calculated risk in the knowledge that she is wrong but likely not to be caught out. We have found that Asian mothers make a conscious decision on the grounds of the child's best interests which generally speaking, is best served by not exposing him to rain, cold and traffic. Health workers have the unpleasant task of explaining the law and its repercussions in the event of an accident. The dangers of using older children as baby-sitters for their young siblings must also be mentioned, including the stress occasioned to the child left in charge who, unless she is exceptionally mature, is ill-equipped to deal with an emergency and too young to cope with the responsibility placed upon her. There are also risks attached to pre-adolescents escorting younger children to and from nursery or infant schools. Nursery schools usually have very strict rules about releasing children to anyone other than a designated adult but staff may not always notice how a child arrives in the morning. Infant school children are less closely monitored but are still young enough to need adult supervision when crossing the road. Although the health worker's advice is proscriptive it can be tempered with reassurances that, provided young children are suitably dressed, most weather conditions do not adversely affect health and there are positive benefits for mother and children in venturing out of doors. Car owners have an advantage over pedestrians but they may also be glad of advice concerning the safety of children in transit.

Electrical equipment such as washing machines, televisions and space heaters may be novelties for the newly-arrived family and one might expect a higher than average accident rate. Our experience does not bear this out. Families do appreciate the hazards and seek advice from relatives well versed in native gadgetry. Probably the greatest danger comes from those goods bought second-hand from a less than honest dealer who has exploited his customer's unfamiliarity with his merchandise by selling him faulty goods.

Medicines are an inevitable concommitant of family life and unless they are taken as directed by the person for whom they were prescribed and have been stored in a locked cupboard, accidental poisoning is a distinct possibility. People whose first language is English often have difficulty in recalling the doctor's instructions when drugs are labelled 'to be taken as directed' so it is not hard to imagine the bewilderment of those with communication problems. A typical example is of the child with an upper respiratory tract infection who is prescribed an antibiotic, a decongestant and an analgesic: the first must be taken for at least five days and then discontinued, the second is long-term therapy which should continue until the next visit to the doctor while the third is for symptomatic relief and only to be taken when needed. It is unrealistic to expect pharmacists to write the instructions in the Asian languages as few would have the necessary skills, but bearing in mind Britain's increasingly polyglot society, there does seem a case for colour coding medicine containers according to their mode of intake; for example, red for 'complete the course', blue for 'long-term therapy', green for 'take only when necessary', and so on.

In a joint family, several members may be taking a number of different drugs which, unless stored separately, can lead to medications being taken by the wrong person. The warning sign for the health worker is a collection of bottles on the sideboard, some currently in use, others long out of date, and all with different names on the labels. If members of the family are unsure which is intended for who and why, it is advisable for the worker to refer back to the GP for clarification. In addition to giving an insight on the subjective state of health within the family, the presence of numerous medications offers an opportunity for education on the need for a lockable cupboard.

From time to time, a series of tragedies prompts a nationwide safety campaign which is so effective that it becomes part of our collective subconscious. The proliferation of plastic bags in the 'sixties resulted in children being suffocated because they had been using them as toys. Manufacturers printed warning notices and media publicity helped parents to become aware of the danger to the extent that health workers no longer felt it necessary to add their own warnings. This complacency which extends to all the other areas of home and public safety familiar to natives, cannot prevail now that whole communities exist who were never exposed to the original publicity.

Surma and Kajal

For centuries, Asian parents have valued beautiful eyes and have believed that the health and appearance of the eyes is enhanced by darkening the rims with a substance traditionally made from the soot collected from oil lamps and mixed with oils. Commercially-made products compete with the home-made variety and in order to maximise their profits, a few traders increase the volume with the addition of cheaply-obtained lead with all its inherent dangers to health. Only lead-free preparations are permitted for sale in Britain but some brands in the subcontinent are contaminated and are brought into the country by returning travellers. Kajal is used mainly by Indians and is almost invariably safe; authentic kajal is sold in small round pots and is of a paste-like consistency. Surma is more popular with Pakistanis and carries a greater risk of being contaminated. Surma is distinguishable from kajal by its container which is shaped like an urn with a globular base tapering to a thin neck with a wide lip. Because surma is more powdery than kajal, an applicator is attached to the stopper. Workers have been aware of the potential dangers and with the aid of a well-designed Health Education Council leaflet, have shown parents how to test for the presence of lead by sprinkling surma on to a tumbler of water; pure surma floats, any lead sinks to the bottom. Recently, the accuracy of this simple test has been called into question and 1986 saw the introduction of a new campaign under the auspices of the Department of Trade and Industry, the Department of Health and Social Security and the Central office of Information. The new leaflets ask parents to take their Surma to Environmental Health Offices for analysis and it is not clear whether a charge would be made; Cardiff City Analyst's department quoted £22 if funds were not made available for free testing. The response from the Asian communities has been predictably angry and health workers now find themselves in a very difficult position. Clients have long been aware of the negative feelings of many workers to the use of cosmetics for babies, which is perceived as contrary to the native notion of babyhood being a time of innocence, untouched by artifice, values as deeply rooted in native culture as the use of surma and kajal are to Asians. If previous advice has left clients with the impression that workers are motivated by a desire to suppress cultural identity, a request to take their surma to the Environment Health Office will leave them in no doubt. Nevertheless, workers cannot allow their sensitivity to the feelings of parents to prejudice the health of the baby and in order to carry conviction that their advice does not imply criticism of the custom, they will need the help of the Asian communities. A joint approach from health worker and a respected member of the community could convince parents of the need for either testing or changing to a British-made hypo-allergenic cosmetic without threatening cherished beliefs. There is no evidence that the use of lead-free cosmetics has any harmful effects.

Mongolian Blue Spots

Examination of the Asian neonate is likely to reveal areas of blue pigmentation on various parts of the body. These are mongolian blue spots and are present on most dark-skinned people. The commonest site is the sacral region but they can be found anywhere except on the face. They have no clinical significance but their presence and exact location should always be recorded because they are easily mistaken for bruising; case conferences have been convened to protect children who appeared to have been the subject of severe beatings when all they had were blue spots. No doubt the workers involved felt a little foolish but one can scarcely imagine the feelings of the parents and child under suspicion of non-accidental injury.

Head Shaving

Moslem babies are required to have all their hair shaved during the first weeks of life. Although Islam demands only one shave, some mothers repeat the process several times because they believe that it promotes the growth of strong, healthy hair. In order to protect the baby from heat loss, a bonnet is always worn until there is adequate regrowth. Repeated shaving can produce eczematous rashes in babies with dry, sensitive skins. Hindu boys have their heads shaved three times in the first five years of life. Sikhs never cut their children's hair. The head is treated with respect and a friendly pat or ruffling of the hair, used as an affectionate gesture by natives, might cause offence to Asian parents.

Circumcision

Islam requires the circumcision of all male children before they reach puberty. Unlike Judaism, this is not a task performed by the religious leader and, although in some areas the Rabbi circumcises Moslem babies in addition to his own flock, most parents look to the medical profession for help.

National Health Service facilities vary according to the policy of local paediatric departments. Those with long waiting lists of children awaiting 'cold' surgery to relieve them of disabling conditions are unlikely to offer more than a very long wait on the non-urgent list. Some refuse to accept cases on anything other than medical grounds. Others, with ample day-case facilities, may feel that a low-cost operation of this nature can be offered without prejudicing ill children.

The alternatives are surgery undertaken privately by a consultant surgeon which is beyond the means of most parents, or utilising the services of a less-highly-qualified doctor who specialises in this type of operation. Where there is a sizeable Moslem population there is likely to be a doctor, possibly a G P, who will circumcise for a moderate fee. This same person may offer a peripatetic service, travelling from city to city, leaving behind a trail of little boys minus their foreskins. Most children are circumcised before the age of two and they recover remarkably quickly with none of the acute discomfort that afflicts older boys. Sutures used are of the dissolving type and mothers are well briefed in aftercare.

Female circumcision is not practised among Moslems from the subcontinent.

References

Black J (1986) *Paediatrics Among Ethnic Minorities.* London: British Medical Association

Bondestam M (1985) Subclinical trace element deficiency in children with undue susceptibility to infections. *Acta Paediatrica Scandinavica,* **74**, 512–520

Campbell I (1981) *The Problem of Tuberculosis in Infants – Report of a Symposium on the Health Needs of Ethnic Groups.* South Glamorgan Health Authority

Ehrhardt P (1986) Iron deficiency in young Bradford children from different ethnic groups. *British Medical Journal,* **292**, 90–93

Grindulis H (1984) Tuberculin response two years after BCG vaccination at birth. *Archives of Disease in Childhood,* **59**, 614–619

Hadfield J (1986) Sensitivity of neonates to tuberculin after BCG vaccination. *British Medical Journal,* **292**, 990–991

Henley A (1979) *Asian Patients in Hospital and at Home.* London: King's Fund

Jivani S (1978) The practices of infant feeding among Asian immigrants. *Archives of Disease in Childhood,* **53**, 69–73

Meadows N (1986) Screening for intrauterine growth retardation using ratio of mid-arm circumference to occipitofrontal circumference. *British Medical Journal,* **292**, 1039–40

Recommended Reading

Black J (1986) *Paediatrics Among Ethnic Minorities.* London: British Medical Association. Chapters on Asians: describes the diseases that most commonly affect Asian children but without implying 'victim blame'

Chapter 5

CHILDHOOD

The links forged between the family and the community health services during pregnancy and infancy are maintained throughout the pre-school years. The theme of this chapter is the health worker's continued endorsement of the family's chosen lifestyle but with the additional obligation to offer those aspects of native culture which will enhance health and quality of life without diminishing the family's own identity. The needs of the young child emerging from a background of immutable values into a seemingly amorphous western culture will be examined, together with suggestions on ways in which to present services aimed at maximising health and development.

Diet Revisited

In the affluent West, the consumption of food has gone far beyond the adequate intake of nutrients. The food industry must continually expand in order to survive and it is no longer enough to provide for 'needs' – successful marketing depends on the exploitation of 'wants'. Almost lost amidst the welter of commercial advertising is the message of the health educators which attempts to promote healthy eating patterns but starts from the premise that most people are carnivores and unaffected by religious taboos. Wooed by both sides is the consumer but she is also governed by her economic circumstances, her own perceptions and the likes and dislikes of her family. The results of this unequal triangle are to be found on the nation's dinner plates.

For families of the subcontinent it was never thus. The food consumed is that which is seasonally available, usually grown or reared on family land or purchased from local traders. Religious beliefs determine what is eaten and when; cooking methods are those which have evolved over centuries. Only wealthy families are able to afford expensive imported food; the majority are not spoiled for choice and are therefore denied the freedom to select the wrong dietary option or to indulge in gourmandising. The nutrition-related diseases of the subcontinent stem from an inadequate intake of the 'right' foods, in the West, they result from too much of all foods, 'right' or 'wrong'.

Very few generalisations can be made about Asian eating habits and the concept of a typical Asian meal exists only in the minds of patronisers of 'Indian' restaurants. History, geography, climate, religion and family tradition combine to preserve culinary variations as diverse as any to be found in Europe. There are similarities in the way food is presented; whereas natives traditionally eat from a plate containing meat, potatoes and at least one other vegetable, followed by a pudding, Asians help themselves from a variety of central dishes, using the fingers of the right hand to convey the food from plate to mouth. Men are often fed first, women and children waiting until they have finished before commencing their own meal. Young children may be fed directly from the mother's plate, omitting the hotly spiced foods. Fresh fruit is the usual desert but on special occasions, halvas – sweets made with milk, sugar, nuts and spices – are served. The main meal is eaten in the cool of the evening, the hot daytime temperatures demand the intake of plenty of fluids but little in the way of food.

Asians in Britain may experience some difficulty in following traditional eating patterns. Most foods are available but perishable fruit and vegetables are very expensive to import. Advertising is also a potent force for change, especially in families with older children, and women may be persuaded to try some of the products which, if the media are to be believed, are an essential part of the good life. Health workers, unsure of the nutritional value of Asian foods, may persist in recommending that which is familiar to them, implying that families should adopt native eating habits because they are 'better'. Mares (1985) quotes a health visitor speaking about an Asian mother, 'She's very good. She gives her children English food'.

The healthy toddler, having graduated from bottles and strained dinners to full membership of family mealtimes, is living proof of his mother's skills in child care and an essential component of the ideal family stereotype. Small wonder that the nonconforming child who turns every meal into a pitched battle is seen as a reflection of his mother's inadequacies. But the facts are that few mothers do not experience some difficulty when feeding their young children, whether occasioned by a natural lack of interest in food, a desire on the child's part to seek attention or just poor management. When confronted by a problem eater the health worker should ask three questions. What does the child eat? What would the family like him to eat? And what should he eat to reach optimum health? Our experience with Asian families is that the answers to the second and third questions are usually close enough for worker and parent to achieve unanimity while the key to resolution lies in the answer to the first question. So often, current eating patterns have arisen out of faulty weaning when the child was not fed on traditional foods with the gradual introduction of spices but on sweetened packet and tinned foods with an over reliance on cereals, milk and sugary drinks. Having acquired a taste for bland, sweet food, anything savoury or even mildly spiced, is likely to be rejected. Also to blame is the proliferation of 'junk' food, which provides empty calories and if consumed close to mealtimes suppresses the appetite for nutritious foods. Carbonated drinks are among the biggest culprits in this respect. Coming from a country where all food has some value, parents may find it incredible that masquerading under the 'food' label are products which do more harm than good. Education is needed on the recognition of hunger and thirst as opposed to a desire for a particular taste but this advice should take into account the custom of frequent demand feeding which usually continues into early childhood. Provided the snacks are nutritious and are withheld before the main meal of the day, there is no reason for discouraging their consumption.

Although adults reared on Asian foods are unlikely to be enthusiastic espousers of native cuisine, they may consider it a suitable alternative for children who have rejected traditional methods of cooking, while women brought up in Britain may resent the time spent in preparing meals and will opt for native convenience foods. Given that both Asian and native cuisines have a history of eclecticism, it is naive to expect Asians in Britain not to adopt some of the native culinary practices. Once again, gauging attitudes is crucial if the worker is to avoid the impression that she is either denigrating the client's culture or withholding information that could lead to a wider freedom of choice. Advice on native cookery should take the client beyond the chip shop and supermarket freezer with recommendations for foods which are nutritious and compatible with religious norms. Cooking methods should be geared primarily, to the conservation of nutrients.

Teenagers may be very sensitive about the type of food that is eaten by the family and here the health worker should take every opportunity to promote the dietary benefits of Asian foods to youngsters who will themselves be parents before too long. Schools could do more to encourage healthy eating for Asians, both within their own catering departments so that acceptable meal choices are available for Asian pupils, and through the teaching of cookery which is a curriculum subject in most secondary schools but which could be broadened from its rather narrow base of victoria sponges and jam tarts, to include chapatis and samosas. The Asian girls will have been taught how to make them by their mothers but would benefit from the demystification and increased acceptance of Asian foods.

One group who may experience considerable difficulty in avoiding 'junk' foods are those in the grocery trade whose profit margins depend on sales of confectionery, soft drinks and non-nutritious snack foods. Most shopkeepers live on the premises and children have easy and continuous access to the goods on sale. The health message has to be uncompromising; 'sell "junk" to those who wish to buy but recognise its harmful effects and restrict its consumption within your family'.

Diet-related Diseases

It is almost impossible to discuss the diseases which arise from poor nutrition without giving the impression that the underlying dietary philosophy of the affected group is flawed and the Asian communities have been hurt and offended by the critical approach of health workers both in the field and as the writers of articles and books. Readers thus far will be aware that only minor dietary adjustments are necessary to compensate for the difference between life in the subcontinent and that in Britain. They will also be aware that the food consumed by a family is only partially dependent upon cultural values, reflecting family purchasing power and external influences such as advertising, the impact of health education and national food policies.

Workers can be reassured that the majority of Asian children are well-fed and in excellent health but our role as community health workers includes not only the maintenance of that state but also the detection and recognition of the abnormal. Without wishing to place undue emphasis on conditions which are not often seen in everyday practice, we should be doing readers and clients a disservice if they were to be omitted.

Iron Deficiency Anaemia Ehrhardt (1986) studied iron levels of hospitalised children in Bradford and found that Asian children had a higher incidence of iron deficiency than the 25% of affected native children. He recommends intervention similar to the Woman, Infants and Children programme of supplementary feeding Miller (1985) which has reduced the levels of iron deficiency in the United States of America and which would be aimed at all vulnerable groups irrespective of ethnic origin. De Lobo (1978), in contrast, suggests that anaemia is an exclusively Asian problem and calls for the screening of all Asian three-year-olds at child health clinics. Apart from the practical considerations, few health workers would be happy to participate in such a blatantly discriminatory screening programme and would prefer to reserve haemoglobin testing for the children about whom parents and workers are concerned. On the preventive front workers can advise on the intake of iron bearing food, remembering that although meat is eaten by Moslems, Sikhs and a few Hindus, the quantities eaten at each meal are less than would be found on a native plate, and that, therefore, other sources must also be recommended. Moslems, Sikhs and male Hindus eat eggs but these may not always be given to Hindu girls as they are considered to be too 'hot'. Green-leafed vegetables are part of all Asian diets, many families with gardens growing their own. Children often enjoy the popular breakfast cereals and these should not be discouraged as most are fortified with iron and vitamins, and provide approximately a sixth of daily iron needs.

Rickets Rickets has been discussed in an earlier chapter but is reintroduced here because workers need to recognise the early signs in the few children they may encounter who are suffering from the condition. Classically, rickets does not develop before the second year of life; the cardinal signs are bowing of the legs and thickening of the growing ends of the long bones of the arms and legs. The child may complain of pain and experience difficulty in walking. Treatment is by giving carefully measured doses of vitamin D. Prevention includes taking multivitamins until the child is at least five years of age and the recommendation of dietary sources of vitamin D that are acceptable such as vegetable-only margarines, eggs, evaporated milk and fortified breakfast cereals. Although the fish eaten by Bangladeshis is rich in vitamin D, it is not considered suitable for young children because it has too many bones and is often salted for preservation. Workers could recommend sardines and pilchards which are similar to the fish of Bangladesh but without its disadvantages.

The Stop Rickets Campaign has been severely criticised for its allegedly racist approach which implies failure on the part of Asians to adapt their diet to compensate for the lack of sunlight in Britain, forgetting that were it not for the fortification of foods popular with natives, rickets would be endemic among all the less-affluent members of society, as it was in the early years of this century. While the campaign could be used by racist groups to discredit the Asian communities, it has been of benefit to health workers by focusing their attention on a condition which had hitherto been neglected. Provided that dietary information is given factually and non-judgementally, families should not be in the least offended and will accept the message in the spirit in which it has been given.

Restricted Growth Jivani (1978) notes a reduction in growth by the first birthday if weaning has been nutritionally inadequate. After the age of two there is partial 'catch up' growth but insufficient for the attainment of full growth potential. Growth is a matter of concern for Asian parents who do not want their children to be at a physical disadvantage compared with their native peers and they will seek help from health workers if they feel that one or all of their children are small for their age. Black (1985) suggests a referral to a growth clinic when all other causes have been eliminated. Although treatment may not be possible, at least the parent can be reassured that there is nothing radically wrong. Protein deficiency is not likely to be a cause of small stature in most young children because the recommended intake of 35–40 g for the preschool child will largely be supplied by the high intake of milk. Small children who refuse milk should have their diets checked to ensure that alternative sources of protein are being given.

Dental Disease Dental caries do not appear to be a serious problem in the subcontinent and workers will envy the almost perfect dental health of recent immigrants. Sadly, this state of affairs does not last. Williams (1981) reviewed studies carried out in Britain during the decades since mass immigration which showed Asian children enjoying superior dental health compared with natives in the 'sixties, a similar rate of decay in 1970, but by 1972 the position was reversed with the teeth of Asian children needing more treatment than those of the natives. We have visited a number of families in which one child has had all his milk teeth extracted before the age of four. The most likely cause of dental caries in a population hitherto unscathed must be dietary, probably the increased consumption of refined sugars and the way in which they are consumed. Bottles are used for drinking by two, three and even four-year-olds and, as we have shown, are likely to contain a variety of sweetened drinks. Parents are usually bewildered and guilt-ridden when the extent of the decay is made known to them. Workers should share some of that guilt because, clearly, we have not been very effective in our health education.

The means of prevention are obvious; reduce sugary snacks to a minimum, never give sweetened drinks via a bottle and encourage the use of a cup at the earliest opportunity and, if possible, retain the eating habits of the subcontinent. Health workers should check mouths for early signs of decay and encourage early and regular attendance at the dentist.

Eczema, Asthma and Allergies An anxiety commonly voiced by parents concerns skin conditions, in particular, eczema. There is no evidence to show that Asian children are more prone to eczema than their native fellows but we have seen a number of sufferers in our own practices. It is possible to postulate a number of theories but impossible to substantiate them. Nevertheless, it is a reasonable assumption that changes in dietary habit, exposure to urban pollution, the use of unfamiliar detergents, the need to cover the skin with more clothing (much of it synthetic) in order to keep warm, and western heating methods could all be implicated in skin problems of varying severity. The advice on amelioration and prevention is the same for all skin sufferers but parents of children who have been prescribed hydrocortisone-based ointments need reminding that they should be used very sparingly. Prolonged use can cause depigmentation in dark-skinned children.

Difficulties may be experienced if the eczema is attributed to a food allergy and treatment includes an exclusion diet. Although advice will have been given by a dietician at the outpatient department, it is the health visitor who has the task of translating the diet sheet into a nutritionally adequate and culturally acceptable range of foods. Lactose-free diets are especially hard to follow because cow's milk is present in so many products, both Asian and native, and unless parents are able to read English, listed ingredients cannot be scrutinised for milk content. Specialists should be almost certain that milk is the culprit before subjecting families to the stress of a major change in eating habits and in very severe cases it may be the lesser of two evils to admit the child to hospital where an exclusion diet can be given under controlled conditions.

Some parents are being advised to avoid certain food additives, not only for skin conditions but also for asthma, hyperactivity and behavioural problems. This is a controversial issue, with some workers firmly convinced that a number of additives are at the root of many a disease while others dismiss the exponents of these theories as cranks and charlatans. As food additives are almost exclusively a feature of western processed foods, the safest advice is for families to adhere to the diet of the subcontinent.

As with eczema, the prevalence of asthma is difficult to estimate although de Lobo (1978) claims that it is higher among British Asians than in the native population and among those living in the subcontinent. Respiratory tract infections are likely to affect newly-arrived families with little or no immunity to native viruses and the early months of settlement are marked by an almost continuous stream of coughs and colds.

Children in Hospital

Only a minority of families manage to survive the childhood years without at least one young member being admitted to hospital and despite the high standard of care and the usually successful outcome, it is an experience few would wish to repeat. Hospitals in the subcontinent rely heavily on relatives to provide basic care, a concept which is now accepted by paediatric staff as being beneficial to patients and preferable to the rigid attitudes which excluded families from any involvement with the sick child other than during the limited visiting times. Open visiting may be a boon to the patients and staff but often leaves families torn between the competing priorities of the child in hospital and the children at home. For a planned admission families can draft in extra help or the husband can arrange time off work but this is not always possible for emergency admissions or if the hospital stay is likely to be lengthy. Visiting does not present a problem for the joint family although families should be advised not to visit en masse as large numbers of visitors per child do create difficulties in ward management.

Ward staff have registered surprise because the mother is a less frequent visitor than the father and assume the reason to be a non-caring attitude. Far more probable is the mother's purdah restrictions, coupled with her lack of English, which makes the choice of the father a matter of common sense. However, the desirability of the mother maintaining contact with a child admitted for weeks rather than days should be explained; this is especially important if the child is suffering from a terminal illness. In order to protect his wife, the father may withold the true nature and prognosis of the illness and death could come as an unexpected and terrible blow for which only he is prepared.

Observation of cultural and religious norms is as important for children in hospital as it is for adults. If in doubt, ward staff should seek guidance from parents who may be too intimidated by the unfamiliarity of their surroundings to protest at violations.

Handicap

In recent years, the needs of the handicapped child and his

family have been the focus of attention from the caring services who have been stung into action by media revelations bordering on scandal. Support for the family, whether from newly-aware professionals or self-help groups, has helped to cushion the guilt, grief and isolation experienced by so many. The realisation that positive intervention can improve the outlook for children with a wide range of mental and physical handicap has lead to nationwide screening programmes so that diagnosis is made at the earliest possible moment, enabling treatment to begin immediately. The handicapped child in South Glamorgan is fortunate in having a purpose-built centre where treatment can be initiated and monitored. Families are offered a home advisory service devised by clinical psychologists, in which the mother is shown how to carry out exercises which will stimulate the infant, and later, simple games to improve motor and intellectual development. When appropriate, physiotherapy and speech therapy are also offered. At two-and-a-half years, the child can attend a special nursery, well supplied with staff and equipment, which leads on to special education according to need. Respite care is available through Social Services which allows families in need of a break to utilise short-term hostel accommodation or a relief family. Financially, help is available via the statutory attendance and mobility allowances, with occasional help from charitable trusts such as the Rowntree Family Fund. Although the prospects for handicapped school leavers are not so rosy, the more able can enjoy life-skills courses at a college of further education while those with greater needs find provision in adult training centres and sheltered workshops. Voluntary groups have made an enormous contribution to the social life of handicapped people by manning youth and social clubs and opening up sporting facilities.

How does the handicapped Asian child fit into this bounteous provision? Henley (1979) describes the shame felt by the family and the stigma attached to a number of handicaps which lower the prestige of the whole family, reducing the marriage chances of family members. She also makes the point that despite the perception of shame, families usually care for their handicapped member with devotion, an observation which concurs with our own experience. Dryburgh (1985) in Peterborough, notes a significantly higher rate of congential malformations in Asian babies compared with natives so it is vital that workers, while aiming at prevention, should also know how best to support the handicapped Asian family.

The first step is crossing the language barrier. Parents need to ask questions about the reason for the handicap, its chances of occurring in subsequent children, the prognosis and whether there is any treatment, and unless they have a good command of English or access to an interpreter, these questions will remain unasked and unanswered. The home advisory service cannot operate effectively unless the mother and adviser share a common language or can call upon an interpreter. Given that the mother will inevitably have increased contact with a number of English-speaking agencies, she should have priority in being allocated a home tutor for English as a second language tuition provided she has indicated her willingness to take on an added commitment at a time when major adjustments are already being made. Visits to assessment clinics place a further burden upon the family, especially if the father has to act as escort; the services of a link worker will assist both family and professionals.

Families may need encouragement and help in applying for financial benefits; our experience has shown a reluctance to apply for DHSS money for fear of being labelled as scroungers. State aid also goes against the grain for people who value financial independence and expect needs to be met by the joint family.

Families have tended to keep the handicapped member within the family circle and may need persuading that nursery school offers benefits for the child. Reluctant parents might be swayed if they were persuaded to visit the nursery and observe the activities. Reassurance should be given that cultural values will be respected and the presence of other Asian children should act as an incentive. The provision of door-to-door transport could prove the final key to acceptance. One snag likely to be encountered is in language development; mentally-handicapped children have enough problems coping with one language which, prior to nursery admission, will have been their mother tongue, and may be unable to cope with bilingualism. Parents may feel that what language can be achieved should be the mother tongue as this is already familiar to the child and therefore the easiest to build on. Unfortunately, few teachers have the skills to teach in Asian languages and special education has to be conducted through the medium of English.

Because the child's progress is inevitably slow and parents have a natural desire to explore every source of help in the hope of a more rapid rate of improvement, alternative medical practitioners are often consulted. These are likely to be the traditional healers, the vaids and hakims whose roles are further explained in Chapter 6, and could entail the child returning to the subcontinent for a lengthy period with the interruption of conventional therapy and, possibly, the discontinuing of drug regimes, which for some children could have serious consequences.

Sometimes the situation is reversed and an Asian family will come to Britain in search of a cure and for the fortunate few, modern surgical techniques can restore the child to normal, or near normal, functioning – but for many, especially those with mental handicap, medicine can offer little and parents whose last remaining hope has gone, need all the help they can obtain in coming to terms with the status quo.

Although self-help groups are unable to offer very much to Asian families by way of support, workers can encourage the formation of sub-groups catering for families sharing a common language and handicap. A parent who is fluent in English can act as a link with the main group, enabling the benefits of mutual support to reach all affected families.

Play and Stimulation

For many years, workers in the field of child development have presumed a synonymity between play and stimulation, labelling the child without opportunities for play as understimulated. Play is defined in material terms, providing the sensory stimulation essential for fulfilling developmental potential. The mother who surrounds her child with play materials is a 'good' mother, the implication being that those who do not are 'bad'. Because Asian parents have not been the biggest spenders in the toyshop, they too have attracted a negative image. One has only to spend a few minutes in an Asian household to realise that there is more to stimulation than the provision of a well-filled toybox. To the Asian parent, toys have their uses but are a poor substitute for adult/child interaction and the companionship of other children. In the subcontinent, a member of the joint family is always available to nurse the wakeful baby, massaging his body, playing, talking and singing to him. When he is old enough to run about he has cousins and siblings for companionship and an environment which provides endless opportunities for play. While older Asian children in Britain may be at a disadvantage from the lack of a large peer group and a paucity of play space, the baby continues to benefit from a high level of contact with the adult members of the family. Asians would be forgiven for thinking that babies in Britain play a peripheral family role, one that is secondary to the all important marriage bond. The native parents who take the baby with them when invited out to dinner are, after the obligatory seconds allowed for admiration, shown the spare bedroom in which the baby will spend the rest of the evening. This would not happen in Asian social life, the baby being an integral part of the occasion. The early bedtime favoured by native parents is designed to give them a breather, an opportunity to enjoy each other's company and engage in adult activities. Asian families tend to share a common bedtime, the young child's sleep being made up during the day when the women are busy with chores.

Sadly, the pressures of life for some Asian women in Britain prevent them from spending as much time as they would wish with their babies and young children. Particularly disadvantaged are those living in a nuclear family who are outworkers for the garment trade who have to spend much of the day sewing if they are to make more than a pittance, or who help in the family business. Parents in these circumstances usually recognise the need for alternative stimulation and do provide play materials. Information about the play value of ordinary domestic items such as wooden spoons, plastic sieves, old handbags and cardboard boxes, is always welcomed, especially by husbands who may be reluctant to stretch a tight family budget to include toys.

Television, often described as the national child minder, is a novelty for most recently-arrived Asian families, who, like the natives, tend to keep the set switched on all day, perhaps not appreciating that for young children, it offers little in the way of stimulation.

Working Mothers

The Asian mother who returns to work has, like the natives, to make provision for the care of her young children. The most natural choice falls on the joint family – the grandmother or perhaps a non-working sister-in-law. Women lacking this support must look for outside help, which usually consists of a choice between a registered child minder and a day nursery, only a fortunate minority having access to a creche at their workplace. Asian childminders, as Mayor (1984) points out, are almost nonexistent and a commonly expressed anxiety is that minders will not understand cultural and religious beliefs, particularly with regard to permitted foods. This is not a problem during infancy when the mother can supply her own baby foods but it will arise once the toddler is eating family foods. If the minder is unable to provide acceptable meals, sandwiches or a thermos flask of soup is a compromise solution but one which may not be to the liking of the child who may object to being singled out for 'different' treatment. The long-term solution is the recruitment of childminders from the Asian communities and encouraging day nurseries to offer facilities for their minority clients.

Mother-and-Toddler Groups

Health workers encourage participation in mother and toddler groups, perceiving them to offer the twin benefit of companionship for the housebound mother and a stimulating environment for the young child. A recommendation to join the neighbourhood group may be appropriate for a few English-speaking Asian mothers, especially if two or more can go together, but for the majority, the typical native-run mother-and-toddler group has little to offer because meaningful social interaction is severely restricted by the communication barrier.

Recognising that Asian mothers would enjoy a break from the domestic routine but only in a 'safe' environment, some community workers have set up multicultural groups with Asian families as the prime targets. The group leader usually speaks some of the Asian languages and can involve the children in traditional songs and games. If native families join in, so much the better, but they must understand that the group is for mothers and not parents, which means turning away fathers keen to participate, this may seem a pity but it is essential if Asian mothers are to be regular attenders.

Some mother-and-toddler groups advertise themselves as 'Asian' and aim to attract mothers from all parts of the subcontinent. We think this smacks of apartheid, with the inference that families are not so much being offered special provision on the basis of superficially similar ethnic origins but that they are being excluded from the mainstream of social activity. Not included in our criticism are groups catering for mothers who share a common language and cultural background where, for example, Sylheti women and children can meet together and enjoy companionship that is acceptable to husbands and elders.

Nursery Schools and Playgroups

Whether parents opt for a private playgroup or a state-run nursery school depends on local provision and the family's finances. Both impose a set of demands which hitherto may not have been encountered. The clock becomes an essential feature of daily organisation; late arrivals and, most definitely, late collections are not tolerated by nursery staff, and parents may be bewildered by this apparent obsession with punctuality. Playgroups usually operate in the morning, commencing around nine o'clock, a time which is the least convenient for the families of restaurant workers who are about halfway through their night's sleep at this point. The undesirability of using children as escorts has already been mentioned, which leaves parents with a choice between disrupted sleep, mother and child venturing out unaccompanied or keeping the child at home. Attendance at morning playgroup will also necessitate a change of sleeping pattern for the child whose bedtime should be brought forward to allow him to have sufficient sleep. Alternatively, he could retain his late bedtime and sleep during the afternoon but this, too, impinges on family life by precluding social activities outside the home which normally take place in the afternoon. State nursery schools offer more flexibility by dividing children between morning and afternoon sessions with the afternoon having obvious benefits for Asian families.

Health workers can help the mother to prepare the child for the first traumatic days in a nursery group. Few children do not suffer some reaction when separated from their mothers into the unfamiliar world of the nursery but, being the resilient creatures that they are, are quick to settle in once the initial strangeness has worn off. The child can be helped to adapt by ensuring that he can cope with toilet needs and is able to ask in English, but beware – a Pakistani child who asks for a 'pee' has not acquired a native vulgarism, he is merely thirsty, 'pee' being the Urdu word for 'drink'! In a multi-ethnic area there are likely to be children from the same linguistic background, reducing the isolation and bewilderment experienced in an environment where only English is spoken. Misunderstandings can occur; parents may be disappointed at the lack of formal education and may need convincing that nursery activities are educative and the ideal preschool preparation. Staff who are unaccustomed to looking after Asian children may mistake the child's carefully oiled hair for a head that has become greasy with neglect. Sadly, the education services appear to be as ignorant of Asian cultures as their health service colleagues, a further example being the failure to capitalise on the cultural heritage of all members of the group. The games played and the nursery rhymes sung are invariably of the traditional English variety, much loved by adults and children alike, and they should not be denied to children of minority cultures, but why ignore the rich store of songs, legends and games that are part of other cultures? A multicultural approach would enlarge the horizons of all children. Then there are the religious festivals, the two 'Ids' of Islam and the 'Holi' and 'Diwali' of the Sikh and Hindu faiths, which have the same significance as Christmas and Easter have for Christian but are rarely included on the school calendar. Most nursery groups provide toys that reflect a monocultural bias. Dolls are invariably made of pink plastic and if leaders are far-sighted enough to supply a token black doll, it is a safe bet that it will be dressed in western clothes. Children's books are becoming multicultural but too often the hero is a white native, albeit ably supported by his black subordinates.

School

Children who have attended a nursery group should make the

transition to full-time education with relative ease. Those without much useful English may spend a part or all of their school day at a language unit until their command of English is at a level to cope with mainstream education. Not all educationists approve of language units, believing that children thrown in at the deep end of English language teaching learn quicker than those treated with a softly, softly approach. As health professionals, we are not qualified to enter this debate but workers should be aware of local arrangements because of their continued involvement with the Asian child through the school health service.

Most inner city schools have been educating children from a variety of ethnic origins for long enough to appreciate the importance of conforming to cultural norms. Children who may experience difficulties are those from 'pioneer' families who have moved from the inner city to peripheral housing estates where schools are not accustomed to teaching children from minority backgrounds and have little knowledge of Asian cultures. Because he looks different, the child may become the classroom pet or worse, the object of teasing and bullying. Children are not born with prejudices but they rapidly acquire them. A number of parents are opting for private education in the belief that the social climate is less conducive to overt racism. They also like the strict framework of discipline and believe that academic standards are higher, enabling Asian pupils to obtain better qualifications which are seen as essential in offsetting the inbuilt racial advantage of native job applicants.

In addition to the standard education provision, Asian children are instructed in their own religions. Moslems are required to learn the Koran by heart, not an easy task as it is written in Arabic which is a foreign language to most Asians. Classes are held in the Mosque or at an Islamic teaching centre and children are expected to attend for up to two hours daily which, for the secondary school child with homework commitments, leaves little time for recreation. Sikhs and Hindus also have a structured system of transmitting religious knowledge but make fewer demands on children. Conflict can arise especially during the rebellious adolescent years, when afterschool activities such as sporting fixtures clash with the period allotted for religious teaching. Most children will, however, accept the burden of learning as part of a religious lifestyle of which they are extremely proud and would not wish to change.

Discipline

Discipline is fundamental to all the Asian cultures and obedience a central tenet of the three religions. Family life is based on a hierarchical system of command and respect between parents and children, husband and wife, and mother-in-law and daughters-in-law. To health workers visiting young children, the importance of discipline may not be immediately apparent as toddlers are indulged and rarely punished. Health visiting does include advice on discipline and most workers expect parents to commence mild correction once the child is old enough to explore his environment and, unless checked, harm himself. They also advise parents to resist the temptation to acquiesce to demands which are not, ultimately, in the child's interests to grant, an example being feeding problems which are difficult to resolve because the mother is unable to comply with advice to say 'no'. Health visitors may shake their heads in disapproval, prophesizing delinquency before the child reaches his teens but, before long, a transformation takes place; expectations of correct behaviour are made known when the child is deemed to have reached a conscionable age, and discipline imposed when conduct falls short of the family's standards. Some of the discipline may include physical punishment which is perceived as the natural way to achieve obedience. As Mayor (1984) comments, some forms of punishment are severe enough to be classed as non-accidental injury (NAI) and as such, unacceptable by native standards. Few Asian parents wish to harm their children and any injury inflicted is aimed at the correction of a fault which unless checked, will dispose the child to be more flawed in the long term than the effects of a few short-lived bruises. Here there is a culture clash with health workers in the front line in ensuring that parents stay within the bounds of the law. Mayor's experiences are that this can prove difficult as parents are not always willing to accept outside interference in what they define as a family matter. Despite this, informal resolution is possible as families are anxious to avoid police involvement and would prefer to remain on the right side of the law.

Leaving aside the minority of parents who overstep the punishment mark, health workers tend to be complacent about the lack of NAIs among their Asian families, accepting the stereotype of 'good' parents who place the welfare of their children above all else. Whilst there is much to support this view, the assumption that Asian communities have an immunity to child cruelty is dangerously wrong. Every society has its misfits and inadequates with a potential for violence or neglect, and the fact that Asian family and social systems are structured to minimise the expression of such deviancy does not preclude it altogether.

Fostering and Adoption

The removal of a child from the family circle for whatever reason, is a tragedy which touches every family member. Asian families have the added heartbreak of knowing that the child will lose his family identity and all the carefully instilled cultural values, once an outsider takes over. Mayor comments on the lack of Asian foster parents which prevents cultural continuity for the fostered child and increases the reluctance of families to sanction the child's departure, every attempt being made to place the child with another branch of the joint family in Britain or the subcontinent.

Adoption is rare for the same reason and now that the disadvantages of transcultural adoption are understood (Gill 1983), every effort should be made to find adopting parents with a similar religious and cultural background.

Going Home

Holidays to the subcontinent are taken as often as circumstances permit; health visitors can expect their Asian families to return at least once during the years in which they hold the preschool health records. In addition to holidays, members of the family may return for important events such as weddings and funerals, and within a joint family there is a fair amount of to-ing and fro-ing.

Health precautions are necessary, in particular, protection against tropical diseases. The current advice as issued by the DHSS recommends vaccination against the endemic diseases of the subcontinent, although none are compulsory entry requirements. One injection will protect against typhoid for a maximum of eight weeks; if longer protection is needed, a second injection should follow a month after the first. Eight days must elapse before the vaccine becomes effective. Partial protection against cholera is obtained with one injection which lasts for six months. A second injection given two weeks later gives 90% cover for the same length of time. A polio booster or, indeed, a full course may be needed by those with less than full passive immunity. Protection against yellow fever is not usually necessary unless there is to be lengthy overland travel and in any event, should not be given to children under the age of one year. Antimalarial tablets should also be given and the recommendation is that they are taken before departure, during the visit and then continued for a month after returning. Travel protection is available via the GP or a traveller's clinic, which is to be found in major cities, and patients can expect a charge to be made.

No payment is required for the health worker's advice on coping with young children during long-distance travel. Most airlines are used to catering for families and offer as many facilities as possible given the limited available space. Parents should see that babies and small children have sufficient fluids, as air travel tends to dehydrate. Having reached the destination, hygiene precautions are essential. The feeding utensils of babies and toddlers should be sterilised before use. All drinking water must be boiled and this advice should include adults who have lived in Britain long enough for them to have lost their premigratory immunity. Milk may not be pasteurised so that, too, should be boiled. Before travelling it is advisable to check that suitable baby milk is available and if not, parents will have to take a supply with them. Weaning foods may not be available either, so a stand-by supply of packet foods offers insurance against a refusal to eat strained family foods. For the older child who has hitherto declined to share the family meal, preferring western 'junk', a spell in the subcontinent could just break the vicious circle and, given Hobson's choice, will leave him no alternative but to eat that which is placed in front of him. Fresh fruit should always be peeled and raw salads avoided unless they have been washed in a sterilising solution and then rinsed in boiled water to minimise the risk of dysentery.

Insect bites can be a misery for adults and children alike but can be avoided by the use of insect repellants by day and a mosquito net at night. Fair-skinned Pakistanis who return during the hot season also need to be reminded about the dangers of sunburn.

Ill-health acquired during the holiday may persist after the family have returned to Britain. Some families routinely visit the doctor for treatment of intestinal parasites whether or not they have evidence of their presence. Diarrhoea acquired abroad, may continue for some weeks unless investigated and treated. Infected insect bites may need an antibiotic. Most Asians have had BCG immunisation; those who have not should be screened if they develop any of the signs and symptoms of tuberculosis, remembering that a third of sufferers develop lymph node tuberculosis, most commonly affecting the glands of the neck (Campbell 1981). The fear of imported disease affecting the native population is largely unfounded; most families return in good health while the unlucky few seek prompt medical attention, thus preventing spread.

The return home brings with it a sense of anticlimax and women especially may react with a bout of mild depression, knowing that it will be many years before the holiday can be repeated. For some, the journey home may have been a watershed and the old life, idealised in memory, when revisited may seem less perfect. Time has not stood still in the subcontinent; economic growth and political upheaval have affected all three nations, bringing about material change and a reappraisal of attitudes and values. It may take a holiday to bring about the realisation that the woman now feels more at home in Britain than in the land of her birth. For many others, though, the quality of life in Britain cannot match that of the subcontinent, a television set being a poor substitute for family and friends, and these women need sympathetic support in readjusting to a lifestyle not of their choosing. Support may also be indicated if the reason for the visit was a family bereavement; couples often need to express feelings of guilt that they were unable to be with the dying family member until it was too late.

References

Black J (1986) *Paediatrics Among Ethnic Minorities*. London: British Medical Association

Campbell I (1981) *The Problem of Tuberculosis in Immigrants – Report of Symposium on the Health Needs of Ethnic Groups*. South Glamorgan Health Authority

Dryburgh E (1986) Neonatal problems in the Asian population of Peterborough. *Midwife, Health Visitor & Community Nurse*, **22**, 26–30
Ehrhardt P (1986) Iron deficiency in young Bradford children from different ethnic groups. *British Medical Journal*, **292**, 90–93
Gill O (1983) *Adoption and Race*. London: Batsford Academic
Henley A (1979) *Asians in Hospital and at Home*. London: King's Fund
Jivani S (1978) The practices of infant feeding among Asian immigrants. *Archives of Disease in Childhood*, **53**, 69–73
Lobo E de H (1978) *Children of Immigrants in Britain*. London: Hodder & Stoughton
Mares P, Henley A & Baxter C (1985) *Health Care in Multiracial Britain*. Cambridge: National Extension College/Health Education Council
Mayor V (1984) The Asian community. *Nursing Times*, 13 June, 57–58
Miller V, Swaney S & Beinard A (1985) Impact of the WIC Program on the iron status of infants. *Paediatrics*, **75**, 100–105
Williams R (1981) *Race and Dental Disease – Report of a Symposium on the Health Needs of Ethnic Groups*. South Glamorgan Health Authority

Recommended Reading

Black J (1986) *Paediatrics Among Ethnic Minorities*. London: British Medical Association
Ministry of Agriculture, Fisheries & Food (1985) *Manual of Nutrition*. London: HMSO
Data on food values useful for reference.

Chapter 6

THE FORGOTTEN YEARS – FROM YOUTH TO OLD AGE

The compression of seven or eight decades of life into the remaining pages of this book may provoke the criticism that too much attention has been focused on the months preceding birth and the ensuing ten years, and that this has been at the expense of other generations equally deserving of well-informed health workers. This apparent imbalance does reflect the current priorities of workers providing preventive community health services, whose brief for total health care has to be fitted around their prime commitment to maternal and child health. The philosophy of earlier chapters can be applied to all age groups and, we hope, will have been of value to workers on both the preventive and curative fronts. The aim here is to demonstrate to workers their potential for enhancing the well-being of Asians in Britain not previously mentioned, and how they can be most effective.

Adolescence

Teenagers receive very little in the way of health care; with childhood ailments behind them, they are unlikely to be frequent attenders at GP's surgeries and having completed immunisation and screening programmes, their contact with community health workers may be limited to health education of the 'thou shalt not' variety – smoke, drink, glue sniff, and so on. To most health workers they are a lost generation, sandwiched between the primary-school-age child who has the benefit of regular and wide-ranging health surveillance, and the young couple expecting their first baby. This gap is regrettable because there is scope for positive health care which could improve life expectancy and health status in later years.

Health workers may enjoy more contact with this age group

among the Asian communities and should grasp the opportunities that are offered. Joint families may include a wide age range of youngsters and the nuclear family may be larger than its native equivalent, enabling the worker to establish links with the older children whilst still visiting the youngest. Because relationships are mainly within the family circle, adolescents are more likely to be present during a home visit than peer group-orientated native teenagers, and are often called upon to interpret for their elders.

There are differences in the treatment of boys and girls. Boys, although expected to conform to the cultural and religious norms of their communities, are granted more freedom than their sisters. They are able to participate in activities such as sport and drama unsupervised by adults, and can enjoy limited contact with native friends. The popular social activities of youth clubs and discotheques are discouraged because of the persuasive influence of western pop culture with its emphasis on 'boy meets girl'. The qualities most encouraged are diligence, respect and a sense of responsibility. Sikh and Hindu boys promise to protect their sisters in the formal ceremony of Tikka or Raksh Bandham.

Girls lead a more restricted life. The usual age for transfer from primary to secondary school is eleven which roughly coincides with the onset of puberty when segregation of the sexes becomes of paramount importance if the girl is to enjoy an unsullied reputation, essential for a good marriage. Ideally, education continues at a single-sex school but this may not be possible in an educational climate of opinion which favours coeducation and as we write, the sole girls' school within the state system in Cardiff is threatened with closure because of falling rolls, leaving parents with the choice between a coeducational state school or a private girls' school at a cost beyond the means of most. Some parents find the prospect of steering a teenage daughter through the minefield of a western adolescence so daunting that the girl is returned to the subcontinent to live with relatives until she is of marriageable age. Others accept the system as it exists but opt out at every opportunity, school attendance being sufficient to avoid the attentions of the educational welfare officer but not enough to maximise academic potential. Attitudes to education vary within cultures as do levels of achievement, a point noted by Swann (1985) who also found that performance in all subjects except English, was on a par with that of native children. The problem of coeducation could be overcome by following Swann's recommendation that children should be segregated for part of the curriculum. Many girls are encouraged to enter higher education and train for a professional occupation and the successful ones are a source of great pride to their parents, making the years of struggle worthwhile. Sikh and Hindu girls are expected to work after completing their education and academic qualifications will help them to obtain a white-collar job among educated women which is seen as preferable to working alongside manual workers from working-class backgrounds. A number of girls do not work outside the home; for them marriage is to be their only goal and the preparation required for a successful homemaker is not to be found in a comprehensive school classroom, an attitude which as we have already noted, has had a negative effect on attempts at nurse recruitment. Contradicting this view are those parents who believe that their daughters' marriage chances will be enhanced if they are well educated – school attendance is therefore encouraged.

De Lobo (1978) describes a conflict in which the westernised Asian teenager rebels against the expectations of his parents who wish him to adhere to the traditions of the subcontinent. We prefer Pearson's view (1986) which claims that Asian parent/adolescent conflict is not symptomatic of a dichotomy between east and west but a manifestation of a universal generation gap. Adolescence is a time when authority is questioned and an identity evolved and Asian teenagers have a convenient peg on which to hang their identity crises. Asian teenagers are more likely to associate the health worker with the native culture they are seeking to emulate, than are native adolescents who will perceive the worker as an authority figure, identifying her with parents and their values. For this reason, Asian teenagers may solicit the aid of the health worker in persuading parents to allow more freedom and an adolescence more in line with native youngsters. While offering a sympathetic ear, the health worker should on no account, side with the teenager, even though the freedoms requested are those which the worker would readily grant her own children. The damage would be twofold: a widening of the gulf between parents and adolescent, and the realisation by all members of the family that the health worker holds Asian values in such low regard that she is prepared to undermine their continued existence by supporting teenage rebellion. Our experiences suggest that revolting teenagers are only a small minority, most are sensible enough to recognise that while there may be disadvantages in Asian lifestyles these are balanced by the advantages, and it is good to hear so many youngsters declaring their pride in their cultural and religious values.

Only rarely do girls reach a crisis point at which they are prepared to leave home. Mares (1985) quotes the case of a young girl who sought the help of her GP and was advised to move to hostel accommodation in which she remained for three days before homesickness drove her home, much to the incredulity of the doctor. If the worker knows that the home background is not pathologically disturbed, she can be sure that the adolescent is unlikely to find happiness outside it. Of course, there are extreme cases where youngsters are at risk but usually the joint family arrange an alternative address which ensures that the girl's reputation does not suffer as a result of being outside the sphere of family influence.

Marriage

Arranged marriage is an emotive and contentious issue, perceived by its detractors as a cultural practice which the 'enlightened' west has long outgrown but to which the reactionary subcontinent has clung with obdurate tenacity. Supporters would argue that those from the subcontinent have retained this custom, not for reasons of intransigence but because the level of marital breakdown is unacceptably high when choice of spouse is left to the individual. Whatever the merits of the two systems, we have found that young people who have observed successful arranged marriages within their families, are likely to prefer the traditional system of parental choice to the risky alternative of the love match, although they do expect to have some say in choosing a future partner, including the right of veto. Bowker (1983) also records a preference for arranged marriages among Asians and makes the point that compatibility with prospective in-laws is almost as important as the feelings of the couple for each other, reminding us that Asian marriages are essentially unions of families. Difficulties with immigration laws can restrict the choice of partner to those living in the United Kingdom and in some areas, marriage bureaux have been set up to help families to arrange marriages in Britain.

Not all marriages are arranged; a few Asians marry partners of their own choice, some with the unqualified blessing of their parents, others retaining family support despite their disapproval and misgivings, while a minority have been disowned because the partner was unacceptable in the eyes of the family for reasons of ethnicity, culture, religion or reputation. Couples who do marry against family wishes may need help in overcoming feelings of guilt and isolation which could threaten the stability of their own marriage especially when external pressures intervene, such as unemployment, housing stress or an unplanned pregnancy. When things go wrong the tendency is to blame the partner for encouraging the defiance of family opinion, thereby cutting the lifeline of support which could have extricated them from their current predicament. At a practical level, the woman who has been brought up to expect child-rearing and housekeeping to be shared with a number of women, will find these tasks far more onerous than the native woman for whom family support has never been a part of her expectations.

Preconceptual Health Care

Preconceptual care has come to the fore as an important part of preparation for parenthood, the target group being couples who intend to start a family in the near future and the aim being to educate them on how to achieve a healthy lifestyle which will optimise the chances of an uncomplicated pregnancy and a successful outcome. A cursory glance at the content and format of this type of health education reveals little that would appeal to most Asian couples; the group setting is unacceptable and the topics discussed, exercise, diet, abstinence from tobacco and alcohol, are largely irrelevant in the context in which they are normally presented. Naturally, workers will not want Asian couples to commence pregnancy in a less healthy state than natives but the health needs of this group are best served outside the ambit of preconceptual care with its connotations of sexual activity. Instead, it should form part of a continuing programme of preventive health care which would include screening for nutritional status and the presence of inherited conditions such as thalassaemia, and health education in schools, and opportunistically, during visits to the joint family. Teachers, health visitors, GPs and community physicians all have a role to play in ensuring the health message reaches young adult Asians whose needs are generally being ignored at present.

Family Stress and Marital Breakdown

Health workers expect to spend some time working with families under stress and affected by violence, and whether they act merely as a shoulder to cry on or as a mobiliser of support services such as solicitors, social services or women's refuges, they can help to tide the family over a crisis or to start anew. Because Asian family life is different both in values and structure, workers may feel at a loss as how best to support the woman who has been physically abused. The avenues open to native couples range from marriage guidance and family therapy for those who wish the marriage to continue, to legal separation and injunctions when there is no hope left. Neither end of this spectrum of options is likely to find favour with Asians although couples should, of course, be informed that they are available to them. As a rule, families prefer to manage their own problems and not to seek outside help; in the event of marital violence the usual course is for senior male members of the woman's family to speak to the offending husband. Family elders do accept a measure of responsibility for the happy outcome of an arranged marriage and expect to act as counsellors when things go wrong. Divorce is the last resort and reflects badly on the prestige of the entire family, affecting the marriage chances of its unmarried members. As Mayor (1984) describes, a divorced wife, no matter how badly wronged, is the object of family opprobrium, so that for most, the status quo is preferable to complete marital breakdown. With all her sources of practical help blocked, the worker may feel that she has nothing to offer, but she is valued as someone to whom the woman can express her feelings, and a sympathetic, non-judgemental response may help the woman to cope with her unhappy situation. It should be emphasised that marital violence is as unacceptable in Asian cultures as it is to natives and we are discussing only a small minority.

The stress associated with breadwinning in high-unemployment Britain is all too common. Those fortunate enough to gain employment may find that their qualifications count for less than those of native workers; this has been especially true for Asians coming from East Africa who, despite their impressive professional and business skills, were channelled into menial occupations well below their capabilities. Mares (1985) shows how few black people with degrees achieve professional or managerial status, and although equal-opportunity legislation does exist, natives are more successful in obtaining employment and in gaining promotion at all levels. Not only does this leave the breadwinner with feelings of frustration at wasted skills and unstretched intellectual capacity, but he also has to struggle along on lower wages than his native peers. Black workers are more likely to work unsocial hours on night and continental shift rotas and because low wages limit access to good housing conditions they may also suffer from sleep deprivation in cramped accommodation, noisy with daytime activities. Poor housing contributes significantly to family stress and as every health worker knows, has a marked negative impact on the mental and physical health of all members of the family.

Families may seek a way out of the poverty trap by leaving paid employment and starting a business, often going into debt to raise the necessary capital. Although answerable only to themselves and their creditors, small businesses are vulnerable to a fluctuating national economy and have been badly hit by the reduced spending power of the increasing number of unemployed people. Taxation has also taken its toll; Bangladeshis relying on the fast-food take-away trade were seriously affected by the government's imposition of value added tax on take-away food. Torn between the urge to put every ounce of energy into the business and the competing needs of his family, the result is an overworked, unhealthy, anxiety-ridden husband, and when the struggle is for survival, advice to work less hard is not likely to be helpful.

Mental Illness

Transcultural psychiatry is in its infancy in Britain and as this is a book for all community health workers, we can only skim the surface of this complex subject. Helman (1984) defines transcultural psychiatry as 'the study and comparison of mental illness in different cultures'. Workers need to know how normality and abnormality is defined within a culture; what may seem bizarre behaviour to one cultural group may be tolerated and even lauded by another. They should also understand what Helman calls 'the language of distress'; how individuals communicate their awareness of their impaired mental state. Above all, workers must be able to make the appropriate response to the mentally ill person if a restoration to normality is to be achieved.

Readers might expect a higher than average rate of mental breakdown among the Asian communities, resulting in part from the stresses described in the previous section, and also attributable to culture shock – the effect of an abrupt and complete change of lifestyle. Bhate (1981) reviewed the literature and found some support for this theory but also a number of studies which suggested that immigrants are better adjusted and less disturbed than the natives. Looking at psychiatric disorders in the subcontinent, he found levels comensurate with other parts of the world, including Britain. One difference noted was the higher incidence of hysterical conversion reactions among Asian women, who were presumed to be behaving like Victorian natives in subconscious protest against their position of powerlessness within their own families and society at large. In a society which stigmatises mental illness, somatisation of symptoms was also common and this would appear to be the case in Britain. As Henley (1979) points out, there is no gradation of mental illness; one is either mad or sane so families are greatly relieved if a physical cause can be found, as the stigma touches all family members. We have found a number of women who have every reason to succumb to a reactive depressive illness, blaming their poor physical health for their inability to cope, and rarely admitting to unhappiness. Because few doctors appear to be aware that mental illness can present in this way, symptomatic treatment may be given but nothing is done to alleviate the cause of the stress reaction, while the endless referrals to hospital outpatient departments for investigation only serve to create more anxiety. Not all community health workers are in a position to differentiate between a woman suffering from arthritis and another whose joint pains are psychosomatic but they may be aware of social and family factors which could help in diagnosis. There is a danger that all physical symptoms will be labelled as psychosomatic and that genuine underlying pathology could be missed; for example, general lassitude and complaints of muscle weakness assumed to be symptomatic of mental disturbance, could be caused by Haemoglobin E disease, a rare, inherited haemoglobinopathy which mainly affects Bangladeshis.

Our experiences bear out Henley's observation that despite the fear of mental illness, when a psychiatric referral is made, families are extremely supportive of their sick member and usually cooperate in helping to bring about a return to normality. Admission to hospital should be a last resort, not only for the sake of the family but because the impact of the average psychiatric ward on the newly-admitted Asian patient will inevitably be negative unless he is fortunate enough to live near a transcultural psychiatric unit of the type described by Rack (1982), in which mental illness is defined in the patient's cultural terms and treated accordingly by workers well versed in minority cultures.

Community psychiatric nursing services have a potential for preventing what Khandwalla (1984) notes to be high readmission rates. He and Alibhai describe a successful community therapy scheme for Asian women in Birmingham which has restored confidence to the participants and reduced their feelings of isolation and confinement within the family. Also in Birmingham, Jervis (1986) writes about community support groups aiming to provide psychotherapy in a social setting. The staff involved were not knowledgeable about Asian cultures but did have qualities of respect and openmindedness which enabled them to learn as the scheme progressed and gave the patients an opportunity to act as teachers. This type of therapy has been termed 'side-by-side' psychiatry.

Traditional Healers

Orthodox medicine forms only a small proportion of health care in most third-world countries. The following table shows the disparity in the ratio of doctors and hospital beds per population.

Country	*Population per physician*	*Hspital beds per 10,000 population*
England and Wales	659	86.3
India	3,652	7.8
Bangladesh12,378	2.3	

(Source: WHO 1980)

In addition to their scarcity, doctors are relatively inaccessible to the rural population and the cost of their services is beyond the means of most people who look to the traditional healers for much of their health care. These healers are the hakims who serve the Moslem population and whose system of medicine is called Unani, and the Hindu practitioners of Ayurvedic medicine the vaids. Their crucial role in the provision of health care is recognised by the governments of the subcontinent who have formalised the systems by insisting on a four-year period of training at college before being allowed to practice. The Indian government supports 91 Ayurvedic and 10 Unani medical colleges. Traditional healers in the subcontinent, as in many other parts of the world, base their practice of medicine on the humoral theory which holds that the body consists of three humours; bile, wind and phlegm, and unless these are maintained in equilibrium, ill-health will prevail. Diagnosis depends upon careful history-taking with particular attention being paid to dietary habits, and a physical examination with emphasis on the rate and quality of the patient's pulse; reference may also be made to the horoscope. Treatment includes adjustment of the diet to correct any imbalance between 'hot' and 'cold' foods which may have precipitated the condition or be delaying a return to health. Herbal remedies are usually prescribed and because most healers serve a relatively small population, they have the advantage of knowing their patients and having the time to listen to them – thus an element of psychotherapy is also included. Charges are made but ability to pay is taken into account and fees are certainly far lower than those levied by orthodox doctors.

In Britain, orthodox health care is freely available to all members of society and until recently those consulting alternative or complementary medical practioners were either rich, eccentric or both. Disillusionment with the symptom-orientation of orthodox medicine has led more people to explore what was derisively labelled the lunatic fringe of medicine but which is now enjoying popularity, respectability and recognition from an increasing number of clients. Hakims and vaids are a part of the British complementary medical scene and have acquired a small native clientele, although most patients do originate from the subcontinent. The advantages for the patients include freedom of communication, time in which to explain their symptoms, and treatment which accords with their own perceptions of ideal health care.

Given that patients are happy with the services of traditional healers, it may seem churlish to sound a warning note; whereas in the subcontinent healers must be qualified this is not so in Britain and anyone can call himself a hakim or a vaid with the obvious danger that patients suffering from a serious but potentially treatable condition could be consulting an untrained person with very little experience. A good healer will always advise a patient to seek orthodox medical care if he thinks it necessary. Some of the herbal remedies could interact with drugs prescribed by a physician which are being taken concurrently and may also contain lead, which has well-known toxic side effects. Because some Asian communities live in areas without easy access to a healer, patients may be tempted to respond to advertisements in Asian-language newspapers offering a postal service; this would not be considered ethical by established healers but could be used as a last resort by those in despair about their poor health.

Community health workers are identified with orthodox medicine which is inclined to scepticism on the value of most forms of complementary healing; patients therefore will not readily admit to having consulted a hakim unless the worker demonstrates an appreciation of traditional healing methods. Should advice be sought which is most unlikely, on whether or not to consult a hakim or vaid, the worker should suggest that the client checks with other members of his community and only patronises one with recognised qualifications and a good reputation, and that he should not discontinue any orthodox drug therapy already instituted without informing his GP. The members of the primary health care team expect to understand each other's roles but if primary health care is coming from an additional source outside the conventional team it is essential that the liaison taken for granted within the team is extended to include those who share the same aim but use different means for its achievement.

Dealing With Racism

Few Asians in Britain can claim that they have never been the victims of racial discrimination (Mares 1985), while many live in fear of assault and harrassment. Health workers have a dual combative role: firstly, they can, by their own attitudes, leave clients in no doubt that racism is not condoned by right-thinking people in Britain and this reassurance is very necessary for Asians who may feel that the white world is solidly against them; secondly, they can initiate action to prevent the recurrance of attacks. Families do not readily admit to being the victims of racism and need to have a good relationship of some length with their health workers before volunteering such information. A little gentle probing may be necessary and workers should look for tell-tale signs such as graffiti, broken windows and children kept indoors during fine weather. Much as she would like to, the health worker is ill-equipped to take on the miscreants single-handed and she will not be encouraged to take the case to the police, their impartiality being suspect in the eyes of many Asians. The best course of action is to seek the permission of the family to report the incident to the local Council For Racial Equality. After a preliminary investigation there would be contact with the police liaison officer who would mobilise the local force to provide extra surveillance in the neighbourhood but without directly involving the family with the police. If, as is often the case, the culprits are youngsters, there is scope for community relations workers to promote racial harmony by working with school and youth groups. At all costs, the worker should discourage any retaliatory action by the victims' own community; this can only lead to more violence. If the harrassment is persistent and takes place on a local authority housing estate, the worker can support requests for a transfer to a more enlightened area.

Doctors' Wives

A group with backgrounds very different from those described so far are the junior hospital doctors who come to Britain from the subcontinent to gain postgraduate qualifications. The need to pass language tests and the rise in medical unemployment have reduced the numbers but they remain an essential part of health service medical manpower. Length of stay varies but it is usually long enough to make it worthwhile for families to accompany their menfolk. As a group, doctors' wives have a raw deal from community health services; their husbands are presumed to know all there is to know about child care and health so families are accorded low priority by health workers, which in practice means that they are generally ignored. Asian doctors' wives need more than average support from workers to help compensate for their isolated position in the community, without relatives or a network of compatriots with whom they are socially compatible, and with insufficient time to establish links with the native population before moving on to the next job in another part of the country. Women can expect little in the way of help or companionship from their husbands who, already stretched by long hours of overtime, must devote every spare minute of spare time to study if they are to pass the examinations that hold the key to their future employment prospects. The family may be accommodated in a hospital housing complex which does reduce the isolation but also serves to create a medical ghetto, cut off from the mainstream of the population. Others may have to rely on the private rented sector which is something of a lottery unless the couple know the locality, and is also a drain on a not very generous salary.

Communication is not likely to be a problem for women who are educated, possibly to degree level and beyond; indeed, some might be willing to act as interpreters or translators. Others will be fully committed caring for young children and running a home without the domestic help that middle-class wives take for granted in the subcontinent. Health workers have an enormous potential for helping to make the family's stay in Britain a happy one; probably the most valuable contribution is an introduction to one of the local contact groups, such as the Housewives' Register, which provides a source of friendship and mental refreshment for women who would otherwise be isolated.

The Elderly

The popular stereotype of the elderly Asian depicts a person revered for his accumulated wisdom and lovingly cared for by the able-bodied members of his family who do not confuse physical infirmity with mental senility. The elderly Asian expects to participate in family decision-making and is valued as a counsellor by less experienced family members; not for him the relegation to a position of no importance as seen in native society which perceives old age as a regressive state – 'second childishness'.

Most of today's elderly Asians came to Britain to join the sons who had migrated during the fifties and sixties but their numbers are swelled by East African Asians who had no choice but to accompany their evicted families. By the end of the century the original migrants will, themselves have reached retirement age and will no doubt, be hoping that geriatric health services will be a little less monocultural than at present. Many would like to return to the subcontinent but for practical reasons this is a dream few will be able to realise.

The assumption that British Asians will continue to care for their elderly relatives as outlined above, is a dangerous one. As we have already seen, housing is not designed for joint family living and whereas in the subcontinent there would be a number of adults to share in the care of elders, in Britain, the burden is likely to fall upon one couple who will find the attendant pressures as onerous as those experienced by natives, perhaps more so given that support services are less acceptable to the elderly Asian. Sastry (1981), reviewing recent hospital admissions for elderly Asian Cardiffians, found that approximately one eighth were for social reasons. Sastry's study also showed no differences between Asians and natives in the medical conditions that precipitated non-special hospital admissions. If clinical needs are similar for both groups, the delivery of health care is certainly not and whether the patient is cared for in hospital or in the community, attention to cultural beliefs is essential. One of the greatest fears of the elderly Asian is that his spiritual well-being will be compromised by cultural violation when he becomes too feeble to insist on conformity.

If possible, nurses should be of the same sex as their patients as it is not the custom for intimate nursing care to be carried out by a member of the opposite sex. If a female nurse is providing general nursing care to an elderly man in his home, she should ask a male member of the household to wash the genitalia and attend to toilet needs, leaving the room while this is being done. Most of the elderly Asians currently receiving health care in Britain have had little opportunity or incentive for learning English, so interpreting needs must be considered. The patient in hospital will appreciate an interpreter of the same sex and one who is beyond the first flush of youth. At home, English-speaking family members can ensure that his needs are made known, although they may feel embarrassed by the elderly person's perception of the health worker as someone to whom orders should be issued with the expectation of instant obedience. There is no place for the jocular patronisation that has characterised the native attitude to the elderly sick person; elderly Asians are most offended at being treated like children. Many will have very clear ideas about their health needs during illness which stems from the humoral theory of disease with its emphasis on balance, and faith in the curative power of western health care will be greatly reduced if these needs are ignored. In particular, diet should match beliefs that certain illnesses are 'hot' and must be treated with 'cold' foods, and vice versa. The patient with a cold wants to counteract his condition with 'hot' foods, plenty of warm clothes and a high room temperature. If he has a febrile condition, 'cold' foods are taken and sponging with cool water is also appreciated.

The preventive health services operating under financial stringencies are inevitably limited in the practical help that can maintain quality of life for all elderly people and their carers, and that which is available is inappropriate for most elderly Asians, which must account for Bhalla's finding of low uptake of services by the elders of ethnic minority groups (1981). Meals-on-wheels, geared as they are to native tastes and cultural norms, are completely unacceptable but home helps, especially those recruited from the minority communities, could be of value to the few unsupported elderly Asians. Day-centre placements are likely to be refused, although a day hospital which promised treatment rather than safe keeping, might prove more attractive. Local authority homes for the elderly are quite unsuitable for anyone outside the predominating native culture and it is difficult to see how they could be adapted to meet the needs of a multicultural society. Old age is a time when the familiar becomes all important and if integration has not been a fact of life thus far, it is unlikely to be achieved at this late stage when adaptability is at its lowest. Asians could learn from the Jewish experience in which a mismatch of state provision and religious imperatives led to the establishment of homes for the elderly in which residents live according to Jewish traditions. Funding is from a combination of personal wealth, state benefits and charitable sources, although it could be argued that such homes should enjoy the same type of funding as a local authority home for the elderly and be run as a part of local provision. It is not too soon for health and social services to liaise with minority religious leaders to determine the needs of the elderly both in respect of residential care and community services. Why not halal meals-on-wheels and day centres attached to the Mosque, Temple or Gurdwara? And why not more four or five-bedroomed council houses so that the joint family can fulfil its role in caring for its elderly members? If the answers include the cost factor we suggest that culture-specific provision is most likely to be cost effective and there is no reason why it should be more expensive than services currently provided for natives.

Death

The customs that surround death are both a means to an end and an end in themselves, enabling the person to die content in the knowledge that to the last, he has conformed with the norms of his religion, and helping those left behind to grieve constructively. Health workers need to cope with their own feelings about death before they can render the ultimate service and if they do not understand the way in which their clients approach death, their impact is likely to be negative, creating distress when there is scope for alleviation. A worker who is well acquainted with the traditional rituals associated with dying is perceived as a source of comfort, offering security against the unintentional violation of beliefs and, more positively, as someone who can facilitate the expedition of essential customary practices.

The desire of almost every Asian born in the subcontinent is to die in his homeland and even those whose circumstances prevented them from spending all their old age at 'home' will make strenuous efforts to return when their demise seems imminent. For many, without any relatives other than British residents or who have suddenly become terminally ill, the reality is death in Britain and this will be the case for an increasing number, including those born and reared here who, nonetheless, want to die according to their religious custom.

Hindus

The dying person is read passages from the Holy Book, the Bhagvad Gita, and prayers are said. Water taken from the river Ganges is sipped; a bottle of water being kept in most Hindu homes for this purpose. Thread, similar to that used for babies, may be tied around the wrist. After death, it is believed that the soul immediately leaves the body to start its new life and as it is the hope of every Hindu not to be reborn but to achieve unity with God, His name is repeated into the ear of the dying person so that he may concentrate his last thoughts on his Creator. Members of the family of the same sex as the deceased wash and prepare the body for cremation which should follow as soon as possible, afterwards, the ashes are transported to India where they are scattered on the waters of the Ganges. Families unable to afford the expense of the journey to India, take the ashes out to sea or to a river where they are scattered by a priest. Because the life of the dead person has been only a transitory phase in the long process of seeking unity with God, mourning is brief. Burial is usual for children.

Sikhs

Sikh customs are similar to Hindus: the Guru Granth Sahib is read and prayers said to the dying person. The body is cremated with the five signs of Sikhism and if funds allow, the ashes are taken to the holy city of Amritsar. The mourning period is longer than that of Hindus and includes a service in the Gurdwara with prayers and readings in the home.

Moslems

Moslems about to die should be facing Mecca and like the newborn child, the call to prayer is whispered into the ear. After death, the body is washed by a family member of the same sex and taken to the mosque where the men conduct a funeral service prior to burial which should take place within twenty-four hours. Some families go to great expense to transport the body to the subcontinent for a burial which conforms exactly with Islamic law, others have to accept the British system which places religious custom second to the legal requirements of certification and in some instances, postmortem examination. Moslems buried in Britain usually obtain a plot in an area of the cemetery reserved exclusively for their use. Mourning for the immediate family lasts for 40 days. White is worn by all three religious groups. We have found hospital mortuary staff and undertakers to be well versed in Asian cultural practices and families have expressed appreciation of the sensitive application of their knowledge.

Bereavement

Bereavement visits are not the easiest part of the community health worker's role but few would deny that they are essential or doubt their value to the grieving native family. In contrast, workers may feel that a visit to an Asian family will be seen as an alien intrusion on private grief; this has not been our experience and we would encourage workers to maintain contact during the mourning period. Workers accustomed to the exercise of emotional restraint by bereaved natives, may be taken aback by the uninhibited expressions of grief which characterise mourning in the Asian cultures. Men and women use separate rooms and are accompanied by relatives and friends who join in the invocations that are a part of the rituals of mourning and encourage the bereaved to act out their grief. Because the intensity of grief is so strong, the worker may wonder whether medical intervention is necessary but before enlisting further help she should ascertain the opinion of a member of the same culture as to the normality or otherwise of the grief reaction. Almost invariably she will be reassured that behaviour accords with cultural expectations.

During subsequent visits the worker may have to take the brunt of recriminations against professionals for 'allowing' the person to die especially if the death occurred in hospital. Remarks made by staff may have been misconstrued leaving relatives with the impression that there were deficiencies in diagnosis or treatment and that had the patient been a native, greater efforts would have been made. Bitterness may be particularly strong in the event of an untimely death such as a child or young adult. Families are best helped in this situation by arranging for them to meet the consultant who treated the patient, in the presence of an interpreter.

References

Bhalla A & Blakemore K (1981) *Elders of the Ethnic Minority Groups*. AFFOR

Bhate S (1981) *Psychiatric Morbidity in Ethnic Groups – Report of a Symposium on the Health Needs of Ethnic Groups*. (ed C Rees). South Glamorgan Health Authority

Bowker J (1983) *Worlds of Faith*. London: BBC/Ariel Books

Helman C (1984) *Culture, Health and Illness*. Bristol: John Wright

Henley A (1979) *Asian Patients in Hospital and at Home*. London: King's Fund

Jervis M (1986) Female, Asian and isolated. *Openmind*, No 20 (April/May), 10–12

Khandwalla M (1984) Asian women's therapy. *Nursing Times*, 28 November

Alibhai Y Talking among themselves pp 44–46

Lobo E de H (1978) *Children of Immigrants to Britain*. London: Hodder & Stoughton

Mares P, Henley A & Baxter C (1985) *Health Care in Multiracial Britain*. Cambridge: National Extension College/Health Education Council

Mayor V (1984) The Asian community. *Nursing Times*, 6 June, 40–42

Pearson M (1986) The politics of ethnic minority health studies. In Rothwell T (ed) *Health, Race and Ethnicity*. London: Croom Helm

Rack P (1982) *Culture and Mental Disorder*. London: Tavistock Publications

Sastry B (1981) *Problems of Elderly Asians – Report of a Symposium on the Health Needs of Ethnic Groups*. (ed C Rees). South Glamorgan Health Authority

Swann (1985) *Education for All. The Report of the Committee of Enquiry into the Education of Children from Ethnic Minority Groups*. London: HMSO.

Recommended Reading

Bowker J (1983) *Worlds of Faith*. London: BBC/Ariel Books
Religious beliefs and customs described by followers of several religions, attitudes to marriage, child care, adolescence and death, of value to health workers.

Helman C (1984) *Culture, Health and Illness*. Bristol: John Wright
Chapter on traditional healers.

Mares P, Henley A & Baxter C (1985) *Health Care in Multiracial Britain*. Cambridge: National Extension College/Health Education Council
Spells out the effects of racial disadvantage on health.

Rack P (1982) *Culture and Mental Disorder*. London: Tavistock Publications. Describes transcultural psychiatry at its best.

Appendix 1

SUGGESTED SCRIPTS FOR WEANING ADVICE

These weaning diets have been prepared for use on tapes translated into appropriate languages, and used in conjunction with illustrations in Flannelgraph form or inserted behind transparent leaves in an album. An additional aid is a small kit containing, for example, samples of vitamins, proprietory foods which do not contain 'forbidden' items, and familiar foods such as dhal. The basic script is suitable for Hindus, Moslems and Sikhs, with non-vegetarian items in parentheses. A few suggestions have been included as a guide to healthy eating for the family.

Weaning – The First Stage

This tape will explain how to start your baby on solid food. It is better not to use doorstep milk (bought milk from stores or milkman) during the first year.

When baby is between four and six months old, more food will be needed with the milk. Do not add sugar or salt to the food, there is enough in natural food. Added sugar is bad for the teeth and makes baby too fat. Added salt is bad for the blood.

Your own food is good for baby and can be put through a sieve to make it fine and soft. Remember to take a little out before adding salt and hot spices for the rest of the family, or boil the food separately for your baby. Baby foods in packets, tins or jars are good. Packets are useful at first because a little can be used and the rest kept.

Baby's dishes and spoons should be sterilised as carefully as feeding bottles, teats and dummies, to protect against infection.

Offer just a little Baby Rice at first, and only once a day with the second feed. Give by spoon: do not add anything to the bottle. The rice can be mixed with a little breast milk or baby milk. Baby foods do not have much taste for us but they are right for baby. If baby turns away, try again next day. Sometimes baby turns away because he is hungry for the milk, so give some milk first, then try the rice and finish the milk.

Two weeks later, give Baby Rice in the morning and a little pureed vegetable with the next feed. When baby is used to one vegetable, try another, just one new one every week or two.

By between four and eight weeks after starting solid food, baby may be ready to have a little fruit puree at teatime.

If your baby is hungry at bedtime, you may like to give Baby Rice then instead of with the second feed in the morning.

Baby needs vitamin drops until he is five years of age. You can obtain these in the baby clinic. If you would like to know more about feeding your baby, please ask your health visitor, or at the baby clinic.

Weaning – The Second Stage – 6–7 Months

During the next two months soft foods can be mashed instead of sieved. In this way your baby will learn to chew, which is important for healthy teeth.

Keep mealtimes happy, do not force baby to feed.

Let baby try to feed a little with fingers, spoon and cup, but do not leave him alone in case he may choke.

Offer boiled water between feeds if baby is thirsty, particularly during hot weather.

Continue with vitamin drops unless your doctor or health visitor advise otherwise.

On waking:	Boiled water, well diluted fruit juice or herb drink can be given instead of milk.
Breakfast:	Baby cereal with one teaspoon of boiled chick pea or lentil puree (or lightly-boiled egg yolk)
Lunch:	Dahl (or pureed meat or fish) with rice or potato Carrots or cauliflower Fruit puree Breast or bottle feed
Tea:	Wholemeal bread sandwich with mashed banana Breast or bottle feed
Bedtime:	Breast or bottle feed

Weaning – The Third Stage – 8–9 Months

During the next two months food can be mashed or minced.

Give boiled water as needed. Fluids can be given increasingly by cup.

Ghee can be made with half butter and half vegetable oil margarine: this will help to make strong bones as the margarine contains vitamin D. Nuts can be given if they are very finely ground. Whole nuts or pieces of nut should not be given until your child is old enough to chew them properly. Running around while eating nuts is dangerous because they are light and easily inhaled.

On waking:	Boiled water, well-diluted fruit juice or herb drink
Breakfast:	Wholewheat or baby cereal
	Wholemeal toast with a little vegetable oil margarine
	Breast, cup or bottle feed
Lunch:	Vegetable curry (or minced meat or fish). Introduce hot spices very gradually
	Green vegetables
	Rice or chappati
	Pieces of peeled apple or banana
	Boiled water, well-diluted fruit juice or herb drink
Tea:	Wholemeal bread sandwich or chappati with cottage cheese or low-salt yeast spread (or sardines or lightly-boiled egg).
	Breast, cup or bottle feed
Bedtime:	Breast or bottle feed

Weaning – 9–12 Months

Gradually increase family food in baby's diet but avoid very spicy food and use very little ghee.

Your baby does not need crisps, sweets or biscuits or sweet drinks between meals. Boiled water should always be available.

By one year most fluids will be taken by cup, although an occasional feed by breast or bottle will be a comfort for a while. Refined sugar in food or drink causes tooth decay, and there is an increased risk if sugar is added to any fluid taken by bottle.

Doorstep/shop milk can be given from one year. This should not be skimmed or semi-skimmed during the first few years. One pint a day is needed throughout childhood, either to drink or in food such as yoghurt.

Vitamins will be needed until your child is five years old, unless your doctor or health visitor advises otherwise.

Your health visitor will be happy to learn about the foods you would like to give your child. She will also explain which foods are important for growing, for good health and during pregnancy.

APPENDIX 2

Phonetically-translated phrases for use in child development assessments, devised in collaboration with Mrs A Roma Choudhury, Harbhajan Preet Ryatt and Mrs Vimla Patel, to whom we offer our grateful thanks.

PHONETIC KEY

Vowels	a as in	'dad'	nasal sound a, e.	
Sounds	ā	'father'		
	ai	'fly'		
	āo	'cow'		
	au	'or'		
	e	'set'		
	ei	'take'		
	i	'sit'		
	ī	'seat'		
	o	'so'		
	u	'pull'		
	ū	'pool'		
	ə	'father'		
Consonants	k	'book'	b	'boy'
Sounds	kh	'care'	b̄	stronger sound
	g	'girl'	f	'full'
	ḡ	stronger sound	r	'rain'
	ch	'torch'	w	'watch'
	c̄h̄	'child'	sh	'shop'
	j	'joy'	s	'son'
	j̄	stronger sound	ng	'song'
	t	'time'	y	'yes'
	th	'Thursday'	h	'hot'
	t̄h̄	'then'	n̄	'nasal'
	d	'dog'		
	d̄	stronger sound		
	p	'up'		
	p̄	'pull'		

	ENGLISH	*URDU*	*PUNJABI*	*SYLHETI/BENGALI*	*GUJURATI*
1	Draw a picture.	theswīr bənāo.	theswīr bənā.	aktā sobi āko.	ek "picture" t̄hor.
2	Draw a man.	āt̄hmi kī gheseīr bənāo.	āt̄hmī t̄hī theswir bənā.	aktā manushaur sobi āko.	ek mānaus thor.
3	Build the bricks (blocks) like this	esei "block" bənāo.	is therāñ "block" bənā.	tumi ei b̄ābe "brick" t̄hiā toyār kauro.	ānijem "bricks" bānth.
4	Draw this	yih khencho (or) yih "draw" kəro.	ih khich (or) ih bənā.	eitāre āko.	āwu t̄hor.
5	Show me your – where is your . . .				
	a nose	āpnī nāk t̄hikhāo.	āpn nək wiklā.	tumār nāk t̄hakhāo. tumār nāk koi?	tāru nāk bātāo.
	b hair	āpnei bāl t̄hikhāo.	āpnīāñ dkhah wickhā.	tumār sul thakhao. tumār sul koi?	tāra wār bātāo.
	c eyes	āpnī ānkheiñ t̄hikhāo.	āpnei wal wikhā.	tumār sokh t̄hakhāo. tumār sokh koi?	tāri ānkh bātāo.
	d mouth	āpnā mūnh t̄hikhāo.	āpnā munh wikhā.	tumār mukh t̄hakhāo. tumār mukh koi?	tāru modu bātāo.
6	What is this called? (What's the name?) –	yih kiyā he?	ek kī ei?	eitāre kitā koi?	āsū c̄he?
	a cat	billi	billi	bilāi	bilādi
	b bird	priñdā	pəñc̄hī	fāki (or "bird")	pankhi
	c horse	ḡodā	godā	ḡurā (or "horse")	ḡodo
	d dog	kuthā	kuthā	kuttā	kutro
	e man	āt̄hmī	āt̄hmī	mānush	mānaus

	ENGLISH	URDU	PUNJABI	SYLHETI/BENGALI	GUJURATI
7 a	Give the block to Mummy.	"block" "Mummy" ko t̄ho.	"block" "Mummy" nūn̄ deih.	ei jinishta āmmāre t̄hao.	māmine "block" āp.
b	Give the block to Daddy.	"block" "Daddy" ko t̄ho.	"block" "Daddy" nūn̄ deih.	ei "block" tā ābbāre t̄hao.	dadine "block" āp.
c	Give the block to Granny (maternal)	"block" Nānīn mān̄ t̄ho.	"block" Nānī nūn̄ deih.	ei "block" tā t̄hāthire/ nānire t̄hao.	t̄hāt̄hine/nanine "block" āp.
d	Give the block to Granny (paternal)	"block" Dādi mān̄ t̄ho.	"block" Dādi nūn̄ deih.		
8 a	Put the block on the table.	"block" meiz pər rəkho.	"block" meiz upər rəkh	"block" tāre tebulaur ufre rākhau.	"table" upaur "block" muk.
b	Put the block on the floor.	"block" fərəsh pər rəkho.	"block" fərəsh upər rəkh.	"block" tāre mātir ufre rākhau.	"floor" upaur (or nīche "block" muk).
c	Put the block under the table.	"block" meiz kei nīchei rəkho.	"block" meiz heitān̄ rəkh thəlei.	"block" tāre tebulaur nise rākhau.	"table" ni nīche "block" muk.
d	Put the block behind the chair	"block" kursi kei pīc̄hei rəkho.	"block" kursi pic̄hei rəkh.	"block" tāre seārer pise rākhau.	khursi ni (or "chair" ni) pāc̄haur "block" muk.
e	Put the block in front of the chair.	"block" kursi kei āgei rəkho.	"block" kursi əgei rəkh.	"block" tāre seārer shāmne rākhau.	khursi ni āgaur "block" muk.
9	What is your name?	thumhārā nām kiyā hai?	their nān̄ kī ei?	tumār nām kitā?	tāru nām suc̄he?
10	What is this colour?	yih kaunsā rən̄g hai?	eh kihda rən̄g ei?	eitā *ki* (forceful) raung?	ā "colour" kewo che?
11 a	Give me the red block.	muj̄ei lal "block" t̄ho.	menūn̄ lāl "block" deih.	āmāre lāl "block" tā t̄hao.	māne lāl (or "red") "block" āp.

	ENGLISH	URDU	PUNJABI	SYLHETI/BENGALI	GUJURATI
b	Give me the blue block.	muj̄ei nīlə "block" t̄ho.	menūñ nīl "block" deih.	āmāre neel "block" tā t̄hao.	māne "blue" block" āp.
c	Give me the yellow block.	mujei pīlə "block" t̄ho.	menūñ pīl "block" deih.	āmāre auldia "block" tā t̄hao.	māne pīro "block" āp.
d	Give me the green block.	muj̄ei həra "block" t̄ho.	menūñ həra "block" deih.	āmāre shobuz "block" tā t̄hao.	māne līlo "block" āp.
12	Pick it up.	isei uthāo.	ehnūñ chuk.	eitāre utāi lauo.	ā lai le.
13	Kick the ball.	"ball" ko "kick" lə gāo.	"ball" nūñ "kick" mār.	"ball" tāre ushtā māro.	"ball" ne "kick" mār.
14	Throw the ball.	"ball" p̄eñko.	"ball" sut.	"ball" tāre ita māro.	"ball" fēk.
15	You do it.	thum esei kəro.	tuñ kər.	tumi eitā kauro.	tu kar.
16	Well done!	shābāsh!	shābāsh!	shābāsh, besh kaurso!	sāru kariyu!

APPENDIX 3

A Concise Guide to the Cultures of British Asians Originating from the Indian Subcontinent.

MOSLEMS: RELIGION – ISLAM

From	**Language**
Pakistan	Punjabi, Pashto Mirpuri
Bangladesh	Sylheti (regional variant of Bengali)
East Africa – some	as country of origin
Gujarat (India) – a few	Gujarati, Kutchi

Urdu is the administrative language of Pakistan
Hindi is the administrative language of India
(almost the same in spoken forms)

Names

Male: Use title and full name.
Religious name may be first or second, never use it alone, eg. Mohammed, Allah. If there is a family name, it is not usually shared by wife and children.

Female: Use title and full name.
First name (personal, there may be two), eg. Amina, Jamila, Fatima. Second name (second personal name or title). The title eg. Bano, Begum, Sultan, is similar to Mrs, therefore never 'Mrs Begum'. As there is usually no shared family name, record the husband's 'surname'.

Islam

A world religion founded by the Prophet Mohammed in Saudi Arabia in the 6th century AD. Believe in one God – Allah. Mohammed was the last and greatest messenger sent by Allah to teach men how to live.
Koran – Holy Book, direct word from Allah, giving code of practical and spiritual guidance. See 'diet'.

Dress

Pakistanis — *Tall and fair skinned.*

Women: Shalwar (trousers), kameez (long tunic), dupatta or chuni (scarf/veil), Burqhuah if in Purdah (long garment covering the head with slits for the eyes).

Girls: Trousers or thick tights.

Men: Western dress. Brimless hat, sometimes. Many are bearded. May wear kameez (shirt) and pajama (loose trousers)

Bangladeshis – Shorter, darker skins

Women: Sari, one end used as a veil

Men: Western clothes. Lungi (from waist to calves) and loose cotton shirt worn at home.

Diet

Diet has spiritual significance: there are unlikely to be individual variations.

Pakistani Moslems prefer chappatis to rice.

Bangladeshi Moslems prefer rice to chappatis.

Forbidden to eat pork or pork products.

Some foods are 'hot', some are 'cold'.

Only Halal meat allowed (blessed and killed in a special way).

Allowed all fish with fins and scales, also prawns and eggs.

No alcohol, some may not even take it in medicine.

Separate cooking equipment used.

Food labels need to be read carefully.

Fasting

(a) Considered to be one of the highest forms of worship, and to give both spiritual and physical benefits.

(b) Helps people to practice self-discipline, and to understand the feelings of the poor and hungry.

(c) Compulsory during the month of Ramzan/Ramadan – 9th month of the Islamic year. Ramzan is held ten days earlier each year, varying slightly in different countries.

1987 – 2nd May to 31st May/1st June

1988 – 22nd April to 21st/22nd May

1989 – 12th April to 11th/12th May

1990 – 2nd April to 1st/2nd May

Abstain from all food and liquid, including water, between dawn and sunset. To break this fast entails a serious penance.

(d) Voluntary fasts on other days of religious significance. Some Moslems may fast as a penance for misdeeds.
(e) All fast over 12 years of age, starting gradually from 7 years.
(f) Exemptions – these are temporary if the fast can be done at a later date, or gifts may be given to the poor: children, the elderly, those who are ill or on a journey, are pregnant, breast feeding or menstruating.

HINDUS: RELIGION – HINDUISM

From	**Language**
Gujarat (India)	Gujarati or Kutchi
Punjab (India) a few	Punjabi
East Africa	As country of origin, usually Gujarati or Kutchi.

Hindi is the National language of India.

Names

First Name: (personal) eg. Neesha (f), Vijay (m).

Middle name: if present, is joined to personal name for polite address, eg. Rani becomes Neesharani, but may be recorded separately in British records. Other names eg. Bhen (sister), Bhai (brother)

Surname or subcaste name: (family) eg. Sharma (f), Patel (m). Not invariably used, middle name may be used as a surname instead. If family name is not shared, record husband/father' surname.

Use: Mr/Mrs and full name, or Mr/Mrs and family name.

Hinduism The major religion in India – 80% of total population.
Believe in reincarnation.
Believe that all life is sacred.
Believe that it is wrong to take life.
See 'diet'.

Dress

Female: Sari over blouse and underskirt. Midriff may be left bare.
Punjabis may wear shalwar and kameez.
Western dress with long skirt of trousers.
Girls may wear long trousers instead of short skirts to school.

	Bindi – coloured spot, usually red, on forehead. Usually worn by married women who have said their morning prayers. Red streak in hair parting – married status or special occassion.
Male:	Most wear western style shirt and trousers. Traditional and particularly for wearing at home: kameez, pajama or dhoti (5/6 metres of cloth, usually white, worn around the waist and between the legs). Older men – pajama and kurta (shirt with high collar and buttons down the front).

Diet

Has spiritual significance.
Strict vegetarians.
Some foods are 'hot', some are 'cold'.
The cow is a sacred animal, so eating beef is strictly prohibitied.
No pork as the pig scavenges and is considered to be unclean.
Hindu man are more likely than women to eat eggs.
Cottage, curd and vegetarian cheeses are eaten but none made with animal rennet.
No alcohol is taken except by a few westernised Hindus.
Food must not come into contact with prohibited food.
Separate cooking utinsils.
Food labels need to be read carefully.

Fasting

(a) considered to give both spiritual and physical benefits, and is a personal decision;
(b) women, especially, may fast on major religious festivals;
(c) may make regular weekly fasts;
(d) may fast for special reasons;
(e) does not usually involve abstinence from all food but fasts vary: most eat only foods considered to be pure – fruit, nuts, potatoes;
(f) some eat nothing until sunset.

SIKHS: RELIGION – SIKHISM

From	**Language**
Punjab (India)	Punjabi
East Africa – a few	Punjabi

Names

First name (personal):	male and female names are interchangeable. They often end in 'jit' or 'inder', eg. Amerjit, Sukwinder.
Middle name (religious):	male – Singh (means 'lion') female – Kaur (means 'princess')
Surname (family):	eg. Arora, Kundi. The family name is not always used.
Use:	the full name for devout Sikhs, or, commonly used in Britain, Mrs. . . . Kaur, Mr. . . . Singh.

Sikhism

A reformist movement of Hinduism, founded in the 16th century. Sikhs wear five religious symbols:
Kara – steel bangle to protect from wrong-doing.
Kesh – uncut hair and beard to indicate spiritual heritage.
Kangh – to keep hair tidy, a steel comb.
Kirpan – a short sword for protection.
Kachna – short under trousers – soldier's uniform.

Dress

Female:	Ornate shalwar and kameez. Much brilliant jewellery. Scarf around neck, covers head out of doors and in presence of unrelated men. Adolescents change into shalwar kameez when they come home from school.
Male:	Bearded, uncut hair covered by a turban.
Boys:	Uncut hair in a top-knot, covered with a small white cloth (a rumal or patka).

INDEX

Abortion, 44
Adolescents, 109–114
Adoption, 105
Advocates, 24–26
Alcohol, 7, 52
Allergies, 93
Amrit, 12
Anaemia, 91
Antenatal,
  care in subcontinent, 36
  clinics, 37, 46
  current provision, 39–40
  family role, 41
Artificial feeding, 53–54, 69–70
Asian Mother and Baby Campaign, 40
Association of Breast Feeding Mothers, 66
Asthma, 93
Audiotapes, 33, 74, 128–131

Baby nests, 79
Baby walkers, 80
Bangladesh, 8–9
Bangladeshis, *8*, 18, 39, 52, 117
Bathing, 36, 38
BBC programmes, 33
BCG, 76, 107
Beef, 10, 54
Bengali, *see* Languages
Bereavement, 107, *126–127*
Bhagvad Gita, 125
Bindi, 10
Birth,
  date of, 40
  expectations of, 36
  experience in UK, 37
  registration of, 64
Birthweight, 74
Body language, 31
Bottle Feeding, *see* Artificial feeding
Bottles, sterilisation of, 69
Boys, 65, 110

Breast feeding, 36, 52–53, 66–68
Breast feeding counsellors, 68
Burial, 124

Calcium, 49
Caste, 9, 11
Centile charts, 75
Cereals, 72, 91–92
Chapati, 72, 90
Cheese, 49
Chicken, 74
Child Health Clinics, 56, 76
Child minders, 10, 100
Cholera, 106
Circumcision, 85
Clinical Medical Officers, 76–77
'Cold' foods, 10, *48–49*, 68, 118 123
Colostrum, 36, 67
Community Nurses, 122–123
Computer records, 64
Congenital abnormalities, 43, 96
Consanguinity, 43
  see also Marriage
Contraception, *see* Family planning
Cremation, 124

Day nurseries, 100–102
Death, 124–127
Dental disease, 93
Depo Provera, 58
Developmental screening, 77–78, 132–135
DHSS, 97
Diabetes, gestational, 50–51
Diaphragm, 58–59
Diet,
  and breast feeding, 53, 66–69
  and childhood, 87–90
  and illness, 118, 123
  Hindu, 10,
  in pregnancy, 48–51
  Moslem, 7

related diseases, 90–94
Sikh, 12
weaning, 71–74, 128–131
Discipline, 104–105
Divorce, 3, *114*
Diwali, 102
Doctors,
and caste, 9
male, 38
wives of, 120–121
Dowries, 65
Dress,
Bangladeshis, 8, 10
Gujaratis, 10
Pakistanis, 6
Sikhs, 11

Eczema, 93–94
Education, 110–111
and cookery, 90
and literacy, 31–32
multicultural, 102
religious, 103
Eggs, 10, 48, 91
Elders, 121–124
Employment, 7, 8, 12
discrimination, 115
and the NHS, 27
stress, 115
English as a second language, 21, 28–30
English for pregnancy, 56

Family, 3
conflict, 41, 111–112
influence, 42, 45, 53, 67
stress, 114
structure, 4
Family planning, 57–60
Fasts, 6, 10, 12, 51–52
Festivals, 102
Fibre, 50
Fireguards, 80
Fish, 9, 48–49, 92
Folic acid, 49
Food additives, 71
Fostering, 105
Fruit juices, 51

Genetic counselling, 44
Ghee, 50
Girls, 65, 110–111
GPs, 39, 46, 76, 114
Growth, 74–75
Gujarat, 1
Gujarati, *see* Languages
Gujaratis, 9
Gur, 73
Gurdwara, 12, 124
Guru Granth Sahib, 64

Hackney Multi-ethnic Women's Project, 25
Haemoglobinopathies, 43–44
Haemoglobin E, 117
Hair,
oiling, 102
shaving, 84–85
Sikhs, 11, 85
Hakims, 98, *117–120*
Halal, 7, 74
Handicap, 95–98
Health Education Council, 32
Health visitors, 40–42, 56, 71, 76–78
Hindi, *see* Languages
Hindus, 9–10
death, 125
diet, 48–49, 73–75
fasting, 51
names, 13, 63
Holi, 102
Holidays, 105–107
Home Advisory Service, 97
Home tuition, 29
Horoscopes, 63
Hospital,
children in, 95
elderly in, 122–123
maternity department, 37–40, 55–56
'Hot' foods, 10, 48–49, 118
Housing, 15–17
and elderly, 124
stress, 115
Husbands, 3–5
and antenatal clinics, 38–39
and parentcraft, 56–57

Id, 102
Immigration, 1–2, 5
Immunisation, 75–77

India, 1, 6, 9, 11, 125
Indian Subcontinent, 1, 36, 87, 98, 105, 124
    map, 2
Interpreters, *22–23*, 25–26
Intestinal parasites, *44*, 107
Intra-uterine contraceptive devices, 58
Intra-uterine growth retardation, 43, 49
Inverse care law, 42
Iron, *49*, 68, 72, 91
Islam, 6–7

Jaggery, 73
Jat, 11
'Junk' foods, 89–90

Kajal, 83–84
Kedgeree, 72
Koran, 6, 103
Kutchi, *see* Languages

Labour, 55
Lamb, 74
Languages,
    Bengali, 8, 31
    Gujarati, 10
    Hindi, 10, 11, 28
    Kutchi, 10
    Punjabi, 7, 11
    Pushtu, 7
    Sylheti, 8
    Urdu, 7, 28
Lead, 83, 119
Leaders, 14–15
Learning languages, 27–28
    see also English
Lentils, 48, 68
Libraries, 33
Link workers, *24–25*, 39, 40
Literacy, 7, 31

Malaria, 106
Margarine, 50
Marriage, 3, *112–113*
    breakdown, 113
    cousinship, 7, 45
Massage, 99
Meat, 10, 48–49, 74, 91
Mecca, 6
Medicines, 82–83
Menstruation, 40
Mental illness, 116–117
Midwives, 39, 56
Milk,
    'doorstep', 10, 49, 50, *70–72*, 94
    evaporated, 92
    formula, 37, 50, *69–70*
Mirpur, 1
Modesty, 6, 31
Mongolian blue spots, 84
Moslems, *6*, 8, 18, 36
    death, 125–126
    diet, 48–49, 91
    fasting, 51–52
    names, 13, 63
    see also Islam
Mosque, 7, 103, 124
Mother and toddler groups, 100–101
Multivitamins, 50, 68, 70

Names,
    choosing, 63–64
    recording, 40, 63
    systems, 13
Nappies, 55
NATESLA, *28–30*, 56
National Childbirth Trust, 66, 68
Natural Family Planning Association, 65
National Health Service, 25, 26–27
Non-accidental injury, 104–105
North West Frontier, 1, 6
Nursery schools, 101–102
Nuts, 48, 49

Obesity, *50–51*, 75
Oral contraception, 58
Outworkers, 7, 99

Paan, 52
Pakistan, 1–2
Pakistanis, *6–7*, 9, 35
Parentcraft, 45–57
Perinatal mortality, 35, 43
Pillows, 79
Play, 98–99
Playgroups, *see* Nursery schools
Playpens, 80

Police, 120
Poliomyelitis, 106
Pork, 7, 10, 12
Prayer, 6, 9–10, 18, 55
Preconceptual care, 113–114
Pregnancy, 35–40
Prematurity, 43
Preimary health care team, 46, 119
Prop feeding, 54
Protein, *49*, 73, 92–93
Pulses, 49
Punjab, 1–2, 11, 12
Punjabi, *see* Languages
Punjabis, 11
Purdah, 6, 29
Pushtu, *see* Languages

Racism, 5, 16, 69, 92, 103, *120*
Raksh Bandham, 110
Ramgarhias, 12
Ramzan (Ramadan), 6, 18, *51–52*
Reincarnation, 9, 125
Rice, 9, 48, 72
Rickets, 50, *91–92*
Rubella, 58

Safety, 78–83
School, 102–103, 110–111
Sikhs, *11–12*, 36
  death, 125
  naming, 13–14, 63–64
Sleep, 18, 101
Smoking, 7, 52
Spices, 68, 73, 89
Sterilisation, 59
Sterilisers, 69–70
Stimulation, *see* Play
Sugar, 51, 70–71, 73, 89–90, 93
Surma, 83–84
Sylhet, 8
Sylheti, *see* Languages

Television, 33, 99
Temple, 10, 124
Thalassaemia, 43–44
Thermos flasks, *see* Vacuum flasks
Tikka, 110
Toys, *see* play
Transcultural psychiatry, 116–117
Tuberculosis, 76, 107
Typhoid, 105

Urdu, *see* Languages

Vacuum flasks, 54, 70
Vaids, 118
Vegetables, 49, 72
Videotapes, 28, 32, 46
Visual aids, 32–33, 74, 129
Vitamins, 49, 50, 72, 92

Weaning, *71–74*, 92, 128–131
Wives, 3, 120

Yellow fever, 106